Help,
I'm Fat Again!

Help, I'm Fat Again!

Crushing the Cravings That Have Kept Us Fat

Faith Solomon

Xulon Press

Xulon Press
2301 Lucien Way #415
Maitland, FL 32751
407.339.4217
www.xulonpress.com

Paperback ISBN-13: 978-1-628-1701-4
eBook ISBN-13: 978-1-6628-1702-1

Disclaimer

THIS BOOK IS not a substitute for medical advice. All information and tools presented come from my personal weight loss experience and are intended for motivational purposes only. Any of the health, diet or exercise advice shared is not intended to constitute as a medical diagnosis or treatment. The information offered in this text is intended for people in good health. If you have any medical conditions, always consult a qualified practitioner before using, or applying any dietary, exercise or health advice from this publication.

The author of *Help I'm Fat Again* is not a doctor or health professional, nor does the author possess a degree in nutrition. The author gives advice based upon years of personal practical application and the needs of her own health and physical challenges.

Dedication

I HAVE BEEN BLESSED in life to have two moms. My birth mother Beverly passed when I was eleven years old and God blessed me with my second mother Juanita who is still with me today. My mother Juanita reared me from age eleven and has been the best example of what a woman, mother and wife should be. I am forever grateful for your continued love for me.

To Torrance, my husband of twenty-seven years, thanks for always being my biggest fan and supporter. Thanks for being the rock of our family and I'm especially grateful for the times you sat and listened to me read chapters to you and for allowing me to express my desires and vision for this project. Thank you for your input and brilliant marketing ideas that always take me to the next level! I love you with all of my heart!

To my Dear Sister in Christ: Mrs. Veronica Greene; thank you for encouraging me, for pushing me and reminding me to never give up on this project. There were times you remembered that I was working on this book; when I had put it on the shelf. Thanks a whole bunch for believing I could complete this when at times I even doubted myself.

Lastly to my mom that gave me life; Beverly Miriam Vinson. I often wondered why you named me Faith. I want you to know that my life has definitely been a walk of Faith and I suppose in your spirit you knew I would need to push through somethings in life while ferociously believing I could accomplish things as I leaned on God. I'm thankful to you and dad for my spiritual foundation and its something I wouldn't trade for anything in the world.

Mom, most importantly, as I wrote this book; I thought of you a lot and could visualize your face as I wrote page after page. Although you are not here to see the woman I have become; I could feel you as I wrote.

I could feel your pain and your struggle. While writing I could remember the times you were physically sick and the morning you passed away. It's those memories that propelled me to meet my personal weight loss goal and to write this book. You leaving us so soon made me want to fight for my own life and to fight for you. I want to let you know that we won Mommy! We won the battle. You're in heaven with no more pain and I won physically here on earth because the weight loss has given me a new lease on life. I am as healthy and vibrant as I have ever been in my life! I want you to know that we have defeated high blood pressure and its cousins!

I say we because when I look at myself from head to toe, I see you. And I want you to know that I will always win for the both of us.

Love,

Faith

Table of Contents

Preface

I WAS MENTALLY EXHAUSTED with fighting a battle I had seemed to be in for at least the past 8 years.

As a woman in her late forties; I was really sick of the weight loss rat race that I found myself in. There were now hormonal changes happening in my body because of my age and being overweight was not helping.

From day to day, I just felt heavy and emotionally disgusted with myself! Yes, I would portray the sexy persona by dressing up and putting on the full face of makeup to go out; but I did not feel good emotionally nor physically. I knew that underneath the glamour of my clothes and makeup, I was unhealthy.

I especially felt old and broken one day while sitting in the doctor's office, because I had to face the reality of having to take blood pressure pills every day. Not just sometimes or when I felt like it. I was told I had to take them every day because my numbers were dangerously high. I was seeing a new doctor that day because my previous doctor had retired.

As I encountered this physician that morning, this was different from any other doctor's appointment I had ever had in my entire life. As the doctor talked to me; mentally, I felt like I was having a "Come to Jesus" moment because I was sitting at eye level with another woman, a black female physician telling me it was time to change.

I felt something, I felt a charge, like a responsibility to change. It felt as if she were my older sister telling me to get my act together! I felt like she truly cared about me and my health.

I had to come to the realization that I was no longer in my twenties and thirties; when I could eat whatever I wanted when I wanted.

As I drove home from the appointment that day, I cried but I made the decision I was going to take charge of my health and this was my last round of the cycle I would ever be on.

The days of eating from the drive thru window 3 times a day had to stop!

The nights of eating sugary desserts before bed had to end!

I decided to get my drive, motivation and fight back! I decided I was going to do whatever it took the lose the weight and get my blood pressure under control.

In this book, I share with you my challenges, tears, and victories during my weight loss journey; and how I was finally able to crush my craving with a simple method that has changed my life forever!

I also teach you how you can conquer your weight loss battle and get you actively involved in the process at the end of each chapter.

My prayer is that this book motivates, inspires and pushes you to change the condition of your health for the better.

1.

Introduction

I WAS SICK OF looking at my fat round belly; and the back of my arms looked like the rippled fatty part of the pork bone that we aren't supposed to eat!

Upon waking on this particular day; my hardest task was actually getting dressed to leave the house. I spent countless minutes standing in the closet trying to decide which clothes actually still fit and which outfit would best camouflage my weight gain. The rolls of fat I could see while passing the mirror, just depressed me. My Fupa seemed larger than ever and the foundation garment that I had struggled to pull over it didn't seem to flatten it at all. The worst of my emotions surfaced when I wanted to wear one of my many trendy sleeveless tops. My once skinny sleek arms were now just flabby but heavy. I felt like I was carrying around a pair of extra-heavy dumbbells. So exposing my arms to the world on that particular day; was just not an option.

My butt had gotten so big... It literally hurt - if I walked too fast. And there was no hiding it regardless to what I put on. Many women revel in having a big butt; but I knew mine was just too big and out of shape. It had long since lost its firmness and sculpted form previously achieved from squats and leg raises. It didn't even stand at attention anymore. It was just this heavy piece of fat that just kinda of drooped a little.

The Battle:

Aside from the battle of trying to find clothes that fit; Once I was out of the house, I battled mentally with what others thought of me. Or at least what I assumed people were thinking or saying about me; especially family and close friends.

Going to church was the worst place of all for me since I was now fat again. See, I had once encouraged and inspired many women in my church to lose weight just a couple of years prior. I even held a weekly weight loss accountability group with them; and on my social media outlets I promoted health and fitness to any and everyone. So, showing up at church where I spent 2 to 3 hours each Sunday was really uncomfortable, especially when I had to stand before the audience. I just couldn't get over the negative chatter in my head of what I thought people were thinking or saying about my weight. I felt as if they were staring at every roll of fat under my clothes. I was sure they were noticing how my breast seem to double in size and that I always wore a jacket to try and somehow minimize them. I even wore little crop jackets in 90-degree weather! Although I smiled and appeared to be unbothered... I felt awful inside. I was in mental anguish when I had to be around friends or family and trying to think of how I would explain away my weight gain if the subject of dieting or weight loss surfaced in conversation.

Inward Shame:

My battle with weight fluctuation would sometimes affect me while attending important memorable events in my life.

I can vividly recall planning and having to attend a milestone birthday party for my mother one year. Although I wanted to see family and friends; deep inside… I didn't really want them to see me and how much weight I had gained since I had last seen them.

I planned my outfit a few weeks in advance, as I usually do because the goal was to look and feel fabulous while camouflaging my fat at the same time. I finally decided upon black skinny jeans that were ripped to be trendy and to appear slimmer in the leg and butt area. That part seemed successful however, the slimming pants just pushed the belly and breast fat up a little further. I was wearing a foundation garment under my clothing that I unknowingly had out grown.

The shirt I chose was a black shear sleeveless top that flared in the belly area. My statement piece was a shimmery rose gold jacket that had a button in the middle. I also decided to add a wide black belt to this ensemble which was a big mistake! I had to get dressed at this event hall just before it started so there was no turning back. Because I was away from home there was no option to go to the closet and just choose something different if the current outfit didn't look appealing. I got dressed and began greeting guest and sorta felt good but not 100 percent because I didn't have a full body mirror to view the entire look. I had also managed to lose my hair brush that night so I wasn't fully confident in the hair department either.

My husband rarely comments about my clothing in a negative way unless something is really bothering him. So about an hour into the party after I had already taken a few photos with friends; he did mention that maybe I should lose the belt because it was magnifying my belly. I was glad he mentioned it and I followed suit. But of course, his comment messed me up mentally.

As the night progressed, I could only think about my appearance. Regardless to what anyone was saying to me; I had checked out mentally. I could see their lips moving but my thoughts were miles away. My thoughts were on how big by belly and breast looked to me and anyone watching me. There was so much negative chatter going on in my head and I was sure I was going to scream if just one more person asked me to hop in a photo with them. I left there feeling exhausted from working physically to set up the decorations; and emotionally drained because of the battle going on in my head about my self image.

The Fat Shaming Experiences

Because my weight has fluctuated up and down over the years… I've also experienced some years of feeling and looking great because of regularly exercising and making good food choices. However; there were times I can recall being told or reminded to my face that I was fat or chunky. These encounters were usually from someone I had not seen in a long time or did not see often and those moments seem to affect me greatly.

My first experience was within my first two years of marriage. My husband's grandmother told me a couple of times when we would visit that I was getting fat. You know how they say it… "look like ya getting fat baby". The ironic thing about this was I was at her house surrounded by the soul food she had prepared and I usually had a plate in my hand.

I think the worst though is when men have the nerve to say it. I can recall a couple of guys on two different occasions that I ran into… blatantly mention my weight gain. See it had been years since they had seen me… like maybe my high school years when I looked like a bean pole in a skirt.

I encountered one guy at a convenience store and he called me chunky. I was on my way to an event and it just messed me up in the head for the rest of the day. The other classmate mentioned that I had gotten fat when I ran into him at a formal event in a hotel. I was in a formal gown that night and had done all I could to tuck and suck everything into the dress I was wearing; so his comment made me feel like I had been punched in the stomach when I simply took a trip to the restroom and ran into this guy! The remainder of the night;

I pulled and tugged on the dress because yet again I let a negative comment become the chatter in my head that was hard to dismiss.

My weight loss had been an uphill - downhill type of journey which means all of my years haven't been grim. I can recall several great years of working out at home, joining gyms, weight loss groups and just feeling like I was on top of the world!

I started attending local boot camps in my area where I was willing to workout at 5:30am in the rain and crawl through mud. I felt like a champion after doing sets of burpees without vomiting or passing out. I also smile when I think of the new friends, I gained from these groups that shared my same goal. I vividly remember falling at the end of my run one day and dislocating my shoulder. I didn't let that stop me though; I returned to run with the group a couple of weeks later and ran with a sling on my arm behind the group at a moderate pace, because my fight and determination was that strong!

So how did I end up here again? How was it that in my forties; I was over 200 pounds again?

You are probably reading this book because like me you've lost weight before and gained it back. You've started a diet on Monday and quit before Friday.

You've probably picked up this book because you are tired of the roller coaster effect of gaining and losing and gaining again. If this best describes your feelings... then you've picked up the right book to finally learn how to lose the weight with sustainable results!

In this book you will read of my struggles through the journey; how the light finally switched on in my head; and how I finally achieved the results I was looking for. This book will also be a call to action for you personally. I invite you as the reader to get involved by recording your experiences, your feelings and goals as you move forward in the book.

It is my hope that you will also make the decision to finally end your battle with food. See it's not supposed to be a battle. Food is not supposed to control you. Eating great tasting food should be an enjoyable experience and yet you're able to keep your weight at a healthy range.

It is also my prayer that you will digest and put into practice the knowledge and resources provided in this book to help you to become the victor!

So before you continue - let me warn you that this is not a feel good - "Woe is me" type of book. It's really time that we face our current health conditions head on and make some changes before it's too late.

A Touch of Reality -

As I typed the last few words; "it's too late"

I am reminded of the feelings I experienced while sitting in the funeral of one of my husband's cousins. I had known her for years and we were actually the same age. It had been quite some time since I had seen her so I was unaware of her health challenges.

As I sat in her funeral, the church was packed with family and friends and I ended up in the front of the church. My eyes seem to just stare at the large portrait of her smiling and I couldn't help but wonder… what actually caused her early death? Which disease took her out? At what point did it become too late for her to turn things around? Why did she have to pass away at such a young age? And watching her young children mourn her passing; it was just heart wrenching to me. I can remember sitting there and in my head… I was apologizing to my body for abusing it… I apologized to my internal organs for putting the wrong things inside of me. I also gained a greater respect for my body that day. While grieving the loss of her, I thought of how she could have lived a lot longer if she had of made some changes before her health decline was irre-versible. I don't mean to seem in-sensitive here but death has no

6

age limit and its really time that we wake up and reverse some bad habits that many of us have had from childhood. I just felt like I was in shock all day; even after the service when family and friends were gathering and laughing. Her passing really stunned me; especially because our children were about the same age. All I could think of was - that could have been me. The experience that day just made me want to do better, to have more respect for my body.

So before turning the page I want you to ask yourself this question... Am I really ready for lasting sustainable results this time? Am I really ready to dismiss the excuses, let go of the weight loss myths and bad habits I've learned in the past that didn't work?

If so... keep reading

2.

Why have we failed?

SO, WE HAVE acknowledged the fact we are yet overweight again. We have accepted the fact that we don't like where we are. Yes, we're uncomfortable in our clothes and tired of dealing with the health challenges. Many of us are dealing with high blood pressure, diabetes, heart disease, chronic joint pain and more. We are lethargic and can't wait to get home every evening to our couches or beds to eat and just sit.

We can barely walk up a flight of stairs or avoid them all together; or even play in the yard with our children. Our sex lives have been greatly affected because we have very little energy to get through the act; or we don't even have the desire to be intimate because it's too much work! For many of us, it's been a long time since we've even seen the cookie because of so much belly fat. The two things that frustrated me the most while being overweight was that I didn't have much energy for intimacy; or when I got dressed to leave the house, I would often struggle to fasten my ankle strap heels. My belly made these task difficult for me!

In addition, some of our men are experiencing ED earlier in life than they should be because of lower testosterone levels which in many cases are related to being overweight and living inactive lifestyles.

As a society we have tried to fashionably camouflage the reality that we are unhealthy on the inside. Some of us have even convinced ourselves we can just wear any and everything we want regardless to how we actually appear to the rest of the world. Many of us display great confidence online with our cute social media hashtags and phrases that supposedly make us feel better about our weight.

While I know we are in a time culturally where Fat shaming is a "No No".

The more we mask the problem with cute hashtag phrases and a "yolo mindset" about what we eat, when we eat it and how much we eat; we are slowly deteriorating our health. And for those of us that have adopted a "yolo mindset" about our food choices; are we are truly being honest with ourselves? Especially when we are alone. Do we really feel fabulous when we take off the waist trainers and foundation garments and everything is floppy, drooping or sagging? Are we really happy fat girls (on the inside) when we're mentally comparing our bodies and pants size with every woman that comes into our path?

What we have to realize here is that there are changes taking place internally in our bodies; that we cannot see when we repeatedly disrespect our bodies with certain food choices.

The visceral fat building in our abdominal cavities can really affect us adversely over time. The fat that is being stored is located near vital organs such as the liver, stomach and intestines. Visceral fat is more likely to raise our risk for serious medical issues such as heart disease, type 2 diabetes, stroke, Alzheimer's and high cholesterol.

We must also clarify that although one maybe slender in physique, that doesn't automatically mean they have good eating habits. There are plenty of people that are thin that may have high cholesterol levels or a fatty liver due to their diet. So let's not buy into the "skinny is healthy" mindset.

Regardless to if we are a little overweight, obese or thin... We all have a responsibility and a duty to monitor what we eat and our activity levels. It is my hope that we first love ourselves enough to make some changes and secondly because we want to share a full active life with family and friends.

The Why-

So why have we failed? Why haven't we lost the weight and kept it off? Why have we set goals that have yet to be accomplished? I will share with you three major reasons why we tend to fail and lets see if you identify with these in any way.

First and foremost, we tend to fail because of **"Inconsistency"**. This was major for me. I simply wasn't really serious about changing my eating habits or exercising. I was truly one that went to the grocery store and filled my basket with a bunch of food that I thought was healthy. Or on the other hand I would be full steam ahead on Monday to change my eating habits and by Friday the veggies began to spoil because I hadn't even touched them.

Or I would go to an exercise class and not fully participate. I would limit what I was going to do or not give it my all because it hurt! I didn't want to feel uncomfortable. Sometimes I felt that just a leisure walk a day or two during the week was enough.

Or how about... Eating healthy one day and indulging in doughnuts or some other sugary food the next day or two because I felt I could reward myself for the work I had put in. While not realizing until later that I was just sabotaging my results! Needless to say the scale hadn't moved at all in the right direction or may have moved a couple of notches in the wrong direction. Therefore, resulting in failure, so I would give up.

So why are we on fire and making online posts and videos that we are starting a "life style change"; and a week or two later we're posting photos of an oversized plate "carb rich foods" like mile high burgers or pizza while dining out? It's as if we totally forgot what we had just announced to the world two weeks prior that got us a lot of likes, comments and hearts.

I'll answer the question for you… **We are inconsistent because we simply aren't serious yet! We aren't angry enough to stick with it… long enough to see change!** Our sky-high insulin levels aren't yet high enough. Are we waiting for something to be amputated before we wake up? We aren't ready to change because the Doctor says we have prehypertension or that we are prediabetic or we're just a few numbers away from type II diabetes. We're not serious yet although some of us have been diagnosed with congestive heart failure and we still want to know what gooey good foods we can get away with eating despite our diagnosis.

We aren't serious yet because we don't really believe that we can reverse many of our health challenges; and have accepted the fact that taking medication is just a way of life for us.

Many feel there is no hope. Many feel they can only dream and wish to be healthier. I recently saw a social media post of someone that was showing the world how thin they were 7 or 8 years ago. Their current weight had doubled or possibly tripled in size compared to the photo. The statement they attached to the post & photo was… "life happens." I could agree that yes life does happens to us all but it doesn't mean we have to just give up and accept it. We don't have to just stay there. Especially if we are still mobile enough to make some changes.

Another reason we have failed is because of **"Misinformation"**. We want the quick fix of losing weight by any means necessary so we jump on the bandwagon of every Fad-diet on the planet.

We will listen to and buy from anyone that is selling quick weight loss results! We are willing to try anything from slim teas to shakes; weight loss pills, waist trimmers (that alter internal organs over time), grape diets and cucumber diets. The latest I've seen is a liquid supplement that is supposed to give us results as if we have had liposuction surgery. Then there's the egg diet that promises weight loss by only eating eggs for 14 days or so. See our false hope and mental desire is to have a bootylicious body like Cardi B or Nikki Manaj's tiny waist line" in just 30 days!

The Quick Fixes Don't Work

I remember in one of my many attempts to losing weight, wearing a weight loss patch on my back that decreased my appetite. Did it work? Yes for a little bit but then it seemed I became immune to its affects. I was so embarrassed once at a physical with my Doctor. He noticed the discoloration of my skin where I had been wearing the patch. He wanted to send me in for lab test regarding the discoloration. I had to tell him about the patch I had been wearing and he sort of gave me a look of disappointment. You know that look when something your child has done that just makes you shake your head.

The problem with these products or methods is that they keep us dependent on them. If you haven't truly learned how and when to eat - the minute you stop using the products and supplements - you gain the weight back. See when using these supplements the weight loss success is contingent upon our continuous use which helps the company's profit margin. Not to mention their increased profits if we can convince our family and friends to join the pyramid of success.

God knows, I was guilty of running to that popular weight loss chain that had me counting my points all day and by evening I was starving but couldn't eat anything else! Somehow when starting these programs or products we are mentally convinced that a fat loss miracle will happen! If I just use this product or wear this waist trimmer like the my co-worker told me…

All the while… forgetting that it took years of eating bad and countless trips to our favorite fast-food restaurants for us to be in the condition that we're in. But yet we expect quick results although we haven't yet made the decision to be consistent with healthier food choices or just deciding to be consistent with regular exercise.

I can truly identify with trying fad diets and being misinformed. My first serious attempt at losing weight was with a local weight loss clinic in my area about 16 years ago. I was given a bag of pills and supplements along with some type of protein bars that were a mandatory part of the program. The workers at the clinic weren't trained and they all seemed to give different information every time I went to check in. And yes! It was expensive. I was squeezing out money I really couldn't afford to pay for those magical results. I actually did lose about 15 to 20 pounds while on the program; but we all know what happens when the money runs out.

Aside from two different weight loss clinics; I even tried to take a popular weight loss pill to lose weight which had my heart racing by day two and resulted in a trip to the emergency room. I've bought the slim teas, weight loss powders and vitamins; and let's not forget the weight loss patch I mentioned earlier. So, like many of you I have tried it all without sustainable results.

Just think about it for a minute… when you're tired of drinking a shake to replace your meals and you're sick of the taste; the container of powder just sits on the counter. Better yet, when you can't afford to purchase the products anymore…What's the end result? Let's not leave out the eighty dollar waist trainer you purchased. When you just can't stand to wear it anymore because you want to breathe; you take it off. The end result is that your belly protrudes back out again; because you never changed your eating habits. We often find that we've gain the weight or inches back without sustainable results. The worst feeling for me was when someone that I hadn't talked to in a while would approach me about a weight loss product (usually a tea or shakes) and would just bug me constantly about buying their product or joining their team. Not because they were genuinely concerned about my health but because they were trying build their pockets. The more people they got to join their team and buy the products, the more profit they made.

Culture can keep us Fat

Another way that we are misguided can be our culture. Our thoughts and behavior about food have been embedded in us from childhood; regardless to if you grew up eating filet mignon and fresh garden salads or starchy carb rich foods on a daily basis.

In my house growing up; fried chicken, mac and cheese, and sweet potatoes were the norm on a Sunday after church; and we greatly appreciated my mom for it. Healthy collard greens some-times became unhealthy when the fatty meat was added to the pot. The homemade biscuits (and sometimes canned ones) along with sausage was just the bomb on Saturday mornings!

I even remember as kids the voices of my siblings fighting over who had the most crust (pie dough) in our bowls when my mom made peach cobbler. And topping it off with vanilla ice cream just made it the perfect dessert! So a weekly cake or some other baked dessert was expected and we felt deprived if mom decided not to bake that weekend.

Many times pumping out these artery clogging dishes even became an unspoken competition between family members or friends at gatherings. We always had to know who made the Mac & Cheese? Because, "I don't eat everyone's Mac & Cheese". Or we would only eat the potato salad if a certain person made it.

I feel the need to clear the air on this one. It's not my intent to bash or blame our parents or culture for the way we learned to eat; neither am I implying they are responsible for our current health problems. As a matter of fact, my mother currently enjoys a meat-less lifestyle. In reality they did what they knew to do and worked with the resources they had. Most of us are simply a product of learned behavior that was passed down from generation to gener-ation. But ultimately, it's up to us to make the necessary changes.

Now that we have more knowledge and resources regarding improving our health; the responsibility lies in our laps.

Another reason we have failed is due to the **"lack of support or the wrong association"**. If we are living with family members that want no part in the changes we are endeavoring to make as it relates to our food choice and being more active; it can feel like we are losing the fight rather quickly in the process. More often than not many of us are trying to juggle preparing a meal or snack for ourselves that will push us further to our goal while making a separate meal for the family. This can sometimes get expensive and time consuming. In some of our households; our family members want the traditional meal you have prepared for them and also want to eat or be a part of the healthier meal you prepared for yourself.

Constantly looking at the boxes of cookies, the bags of potato chips and even your kid's snacks can be overwhelming when you are in the journey to drop the pounds, especially in the early stages of the process. I was even being asked to bake cakes and pies during my journey but I had to become strong enough - determined enough to bake them without always indulging with the rest of the family.

Not only is there a battle in the kitchen, one can also find it challenging when it comes to exercising or being active outside of the house.

If it has been quite some time since you've exercised… it can be a daunting feeling to overcome… to get yourself moving again especially if you are doing it alone. Does the thought of doing it alone stop you from even putting on the gym shoes? Are you waiting on your spouse, son or daughter… to get off of the couch and join the gym with you?

In some households there may even be a jealousy factor going on. It may be possible that the spouse that is not interested in improving their health may feel left out or feel slighted when you go to workout without them. Let's face it, sometimes family is used to the normal routine of you preparing meals and just having a night of television together after dinner. They may not understand why it seems as if you are disrupting the schedule your family has had for years.

You may also notice an increase in distractions that may arise when you finally decide to join the gym or to routinely walk in the evenings. All of a sudden, your assistance is needed more than normal with the kids; or your spouse may want your attention for one reason or another when it's time for you to workout. The girl-friends will seem to start calling during that time of evening that you have dedicated to workout. You've got to get the point that you want this no matter what!

Are you allowing your friends or buddies to stop you? More times than not, our friends are usually in the same weight bracket as us give or take a few pounds. Besides we are friends because we share many commonalities. We dine together, we play together, may go to church together, or our children may play together. For the most part we are friends with people we enjoy and share the same values, likes and dislikes with.

I can recall many times starting an exercise schedule with friends and it just did not last. One person is usually busier than the other or may be more serious about losing the weight than the other friend. One of you maybe doing it just for the socializing aspect of meeting and other really wanting to see the scale move in the right direction. And of course, you always have that one that moves a lot slower than everyone else. Better yet; there is that friend that shows up but complains about their health challenges the entire time. Once the friends drop off one by one, we tend to find our own excuses for not leaving the house to get the workout or walk in.

Therefore, we feel alone in the process and just give up.

We can also feel alone when dining with friends or family in restaurants. Everyone around you maybe ordering fries, juicy burgers and such and their orders seem to make your salmon and salad meal seem minuscule. You may even feel tempted to order something extremely higher in calories just because it has been the norm when you gather with friends and you don't want to feel left out. Some friends (although they mean well); will point out what you're ordering as if you're not eating enough food. Or they try to force you to order dessert. You will find that as you move forward in this journey, you may have to skip cocktails and dining with friends until you're stronger and have established a longer pattern of consistency.

Personally, when dining with friends; I have given in to ordering the higher fat content meal so I would feel good at dinner like everyone else! I actually felt like I was celebrating something when that plate was large and full of pasta or the deep-fried fish platter. In the back of my mind, I would convince myself that I would start again tomorrow.

Before long… you'll notice you've given up again in the area of making healthy food decisions as well as getting out and being active because you gave into the pressure of not wanting to be different or to feel alone in your journey.

The good news here is that… I will teach you how you can enjoy delicious food and include some of the dishes you grew up eating; just in smaller portions as well as the best time of day that works best for your body.

I remember one year taking a temporary job. During that season of my life my focus shifted. It shocked me to see how quickly I gained weight because I was eating from the snack machines and ordering out often with the team mates. There was a great sense of fun and unity among us but the fun I was having become evident in how my clothing began to fit. One thing for sure is that we can seem to pack the pounds on rather quickly but find it difficult to lose them.

Lastly, it has always been a desire for me to not to lose this battle because my mother did. She lost the battle and died at an early age because of her health challenges. She was a mother of 6 and died at 42 years old. I remember at age 11, waking in the middle of the night watching the EMT pumping her chest in great effort of trying to get her to breathe. There was a history of heart disease in her family that originated from her father. While I don't remember all of the facts around her death, I do recall her taking a weight loss supplement around that same time. And we all know that many weight loss supplements and heart complications do not mix!

Most of my mother's siblings also died at young ages and I had a cousin that died after a series of heart attacks while in his teen years. Which brings me to mention- it is vitally important to research your family history. This may answer some questions as to why this process has been a difficult one for you to conquer.

Before moving on, I want to clarify that you don't have to have the support of family or friends to succeed at this. Although support from them is awesome and encouraged; you have to simply have your mind made up that you will be consistent this time. You have to save your own life! If you can't find support from the loved ones close to you... then get support online. There are groups on social media platforms that have the same common goal as you and are eager to get you plugged in. I have never encountered an online group that was charging a fee to be a part. So don't let the lack of support from those that are close to you stop you from moving forward.

A final reason why we tend to fail is we become **"comfortable"** after making some progress.

Personally for many years I would struggle to lose just 10 pounds at a time on my own... and it seemed after losing them- I would revert back to my old habits.

The most weight I had ever lost when attending the weight loss centers was about 25 lbs. It just seemed like that was the magic number... I would stick with it that long before giving up.

To be honest... I got tired of paying the money each month and I was seeing my weight fluctuate up and down from week to week because I was binge eating or trying to see what corners I could cut.

But after many years of failures and successes; many years of starting and stopping- I got sick and tired of the roller coaster. I discovered what really works, what's really sustainable and lost the 50lbs I so desperately needed to lose.

Participation:

In the space provided below:

I'd like for you to take a few moments and write down your own personal reasons as to why you have failed. Your reasons may differ from the three reasons I've listed above.

*Writing and seeing your own response will aid in bringing light to where you have gone wrong and make you more conscious of not repeating the same behaviors. If you need to continue on a separate sheet of paper, please do so as it is important to record your own experiences.

Why Have I Failed?

_____

_____

_____

_____

_____

_____

_____

_____

3.

What's Eating You?

I FELT LIKE I was suffocating! My chest felt as if I was being squeezed - and life was being sucked out of me. I compare the feelings to being squeezed by a large python and I was fighting to breathe, fighting to move forward. I felt empty in my soul so I just ate to feel better; to comfort myself.

See - I had lost someone.

This was the year that My Father suddenly passed away. We had no warning... He just took a nap in the afternoon and didn't wake up.

In the few days that followed; I kept busy and I decided to bake a couple of cakes. I also bought slices cake from the bakery. I even ate the cakes that family and friends brought over to the house; you know that "comfort food". I just cried and ate cake... because it seemed to "fill up" this void and the emptiness I felt inside.

My Father was the rock of our family. No one really made any major decisions without consulting him for advice; especially financial.

Although as his children we were adults; we welcomed his input in our lives. He was a loving, praying man and we were proud to call him Dad. So, for me losing him suddenly caused me to run to unhealthy food choices for comfort. The dense, moist - yet fluffy cake - just seemed to make me feel better for the moment.

While grieving… I didn't think to see a counselor or; to go for a run or a walk to help me deal with this **traumatic** experience. I just sort of dealt with it in my own way which adversely affected my health. It took several months for me to realize what was happening with me and my weight gain seem to just sky rocket over the next several months. My blood pressure was extremely high and I began to notice an overgrowth of candida in my body due to so much sugar intake.

Up until my own personal **trauma** - I have to be totally honest and say that for years I did not really believe that people actually gained weight or battled with losing the pounds because of things such as: trauma, stress, depression or even rejection.

I can even remember mentally dismissing some in my mind when they laid the claim of being an emotional eater.

My preconceived ideology was that- they are just making excuses and can stop eating anytime they want just like me. Well, as we all know… life happens and my personal experience taught me to be more sensitive to others internal issues. It also caused me to dismiss the judgmental thoughts and even facial expressions I had once displayed when I conversed with someone regarding emotional eating.

You're not alone in the battle-

I had a chance to interview several women from 18 years of age to women in their 60's - that have battled with weight gain and found it difficult to lose the weight due to chronic stress in their lives or mental & physical abuse. Some express their feelings of rejection and depression and with their permission, I'd like to share a few of their stories with you. I want to share these real life stories from these women; just so you know that you're not alone.

The voices of these women reveal "what was eating them" - from struggling with self-care to major traumas in their lives that prevented them from really addressing their struggles with weight loss.

As you read their stories, I also want you to reflect within your own life. Maybe it's time to start asking yourself some hard questions. Is there an internal battle you've been hiding or masking?; And yet - this battle surfaces physically in your relationship with food. Who are you angry with? Who was not there for you? Who rejected you?; Is there an issue that has caused you to reach for food - nonstop to make you feel better?

Sherry's story:

I am a 46-year-old female, I have been through many difficult situations in my life. Until recently I never thought about how they affected me mentally or physically. But as I become more aware of these things, I am able to connect them to physical changes in my body. By no means am I trying to use my mental state as an excuse for becoming obese. But there is a cycle I now see and am currently trying to escape.

I can remember being a preteen and hearing people say "she's going to have big hips like her family members, she'd better watch what she eats!" I heard the whispers in passing but that stuck with me and before I knew it, I was a picky eating petite teenager who would only nibble. Very few people questioned why and when they did, I just said I wasn't hungry. Which was accurate, my appetite was nonexistent. That statement I heard as a preteen had me in fear of becoming fat, and began my cycle with weight issues.

In my twenties I had several traumatic experiences such as rape, molestation, teenage pregnancy and the death of my child at birth. However, I didn't notice a significant change in my weight until after my last child was born. I was very disappointed in myself for becoming pregnant once again from this person that only caused havoc and stress in my life. I was barely able to keep a place to stay and unable to work due to my pregnancy. I gained a lot of weight during my pregnancy that I did not lose after delivery like my previous two pregnancies. I always said something changed in my hormones, because since then I have gained and gained more weight. I later realized that all of the things I had been through; pain, disappointment and shame were manifesting themselves physically in my body because I suppressed them.

Over the last 10 years I have been trying to lose weight. I have tried pills, injections, multiple weight loss programs and boot-camps. I only lost a little weight for a little while. It is very disappointing. Currently my stress levels are high and I have been diagnosed with depression and anxiety. I am currently dealing with death of close family members, family discord, career and business stress as well as marital issues. And my weight is the highest it has ever been in my life. I can barely stand to look at myself sometimes. When I do the depression kicks in. I have always had a sweet tooth and desserts have become very comforting to me lately. Then I feel bad for eating them. I didn't consider myself a stress eater before, but its obvious to me now. At this moment... while writing- I want to crawl in bed, eat something sweet and cry. But I know things will get better as I practice self-care in reference to the mental stress, making better food choices and getting in the exercise.

Avis's Story:

There were many years that I felt alone. Growing up, I didn't have a difficult childhood experience but I was alone often because my mom worked a lot and my two older siblings were already out of the house. I felt like I had no one to guide me and I was left alone to kinda just do what I wanted from my food choices to mischievous behavior as I approached my teen years.

I eventually got married and the feelings of loneliness didn't change.

These feelings surfaced again in the marriage because I was physically beaten just about every day by my husband. Living with an alcoholic was a difficult thing to do. He drank because of his own issues and took them out on me in a violent way. I ate to feel better because of the physical and mental abuse I was dealing with. Food was there for me when no one else was. I felt a sense of security when I was eating. Eating what I wanted and when I wanted it was something I could control. Food was not going to fight me back and I felt like it was something I had power over. My weight severely suffered because of just eating at will; eating to drown out the pain. I have come to learn over the years from counseling and self-love that food was actually winning and controlling me. Today I am free from hurting and focusing on a better me.

Shanise's Story

I never considered myself an "emotional eater". Quite frankly, the term alone never really made sense to me. I always assumed those that related to the phrase only ate when they were sad and needed to be comforted. What I failed to realize is that stress is also an emotion and food consumption was prevalent in my life when I felt like I was losing control. Whether it was a relationship issue or a financial constraint, food provided a level of solace that I just could not get anywhere else. I could eat in the comfort of my car and, even if only for a few minutes, lose my train of thought. The past due bill didn't require my attention because I was focused on not getting ketchup on my blouse or honey mustard on my pants.

I gained the most weight I had ever gained and broke the scale at a whopping 410 lbs. During the most stressful point in my life. I experienced my first eviction, had to live with someone that made it clear that I wasn't welcomed, almost lost my car to repossession and ended a five-and-a-half-year relationship with the man I intended on marrying! My life was crumbling around me, but food seemingly never failed! It was readily available whenever and wherever I wanted it! Without fail, when I called, it answered!

I never realized the toll the stress was taking on me until clothes stopped fitting, it became harder to walk long distances and family began to make rude, sideways remarks about my appearance.

It's been difficult to find healthier alternatives to handling stress, but I've become more cognizant since recognizing my triggers. I am in no way near where I want to be, but I thank God I'm not where I used to be!

Getting Help:

Friends, its vitally important that we get to the root cause as to why we have gained the weight or have struggled to lose it. We have to discover what's been eating or gnawing at our souls that we have yet to deal with.

Digging Deeper into the why or what's eating you may require you to see a counselor or therapist. Weight loss therapy has become more popular within the past few years as many are finding that the traditional routes of dieting and exercise are not enough to help one overcome their long-term battle with weight gain.

Weight loss therapy is a form of **Cognitive Behavior Therapy** (CBT) which is an approach to psychotherapy used to treat many issues. Cognitive behavioral therapy helps us to increase awareness, and eventually challenge us to change the negative thoughts that often drive the unhealthy behaviors. CBT can also help us to get rid of the core problem, as the relationship with food is often just the symptom of a deeper issue.

Generally, when seeing a weight loss therapist; most sessions will involve: goal setting, self -monitoring, feedback and reinforcement. It can also increase personal motivation, self belief and offer incentives.

I would like for you to take some time to do some searching within to answer the question of **what's eating you?** Have you been dealing with something internally that has driven you to food? Do you find yourself constantly eating to feel better or to possibly drown out the stress and disarray in your life?

For some of us, just writing it down may not be enough. Or maybe you are not even sure what caused your relationship with food to be detrimental to your health.

I want to encourage you today to seek professional help in this area. Search for a weight loss therapist or counselor in your area so that you can begin to address these internal issues. Our mental well-being; is just as important as seeing the medical doctor for a physical illness. Friends, if you know that you need help in this area, don't just assume you cannot afford counseling. Often times counseling may be a covered benefit on the insurance policy you currently pay for. Also many counselors and therapists may offer discounts or charge on a sliding scale based upon your income. So I encourage you to get the help you need.

If we don't heal the illness within our souls; our bodies will continue to pay the price.

For some of us that may mean amputations because of diabetes. Or maybe receiving a diagnosis of congestive heart failure and having to take medication for the rest of our lives. I plead with you today not to allow your health to decline so bad that your kidneys fail you. Neither do I want for you to live in chronic pain because of poor food choices.

Aside from dealing with the sudden loss of my father; over the years I often experienced major times of stress when my family was dealing with my teenage son's defiant actions. He seemed to be in some type of trouble often due to his drug addiction and I would eat or shop to avoid facing my actual emotions concerning this weight that my entire family carried. See some of the stressors in our lives are not always self-inflicted. Many of us have carried the stress from those we love with every fiber of our being. When that stress is continuously suppressed or masked - it eventually surfaces somewhere.

Today he is a thriving young adult and I'm super proud of him. As my family grew through this process I had to learn how to encourage and support him through the decisions he's made. My family participated in counseling to work through this and it brought us closer together. The most important lesson for me was to learn how to recognize the triggers of stress and divert them with exercise or doing something I enjoyed; vs running to food or shopping for comfort.

It is my hope that while reading this chapter and the shared stories of the women interviewed; that you have been able to at least identify what has been preventing you from losing the weight.

I encourage you to do the work in this area. Be willing to do the work on yourself so that when you do start to make better food choices and begin exercising; the weight just falls off! **I truly believe that once our souls are healed; everything else in our lives falls into proper alignment.**

I want to assure you that -Your life is so worth the fight!

We have got to make up in our minds that - Its just food! And there is no dish or meal in the world-that is worth us experiencing optimal health.

Its finally time to give yourself the gift of freedom to make better food choices and the ability to exercise without the emotional constraints of your past.

Participation time:

In the space provided below:

Please take a few moments and write down the event or experience that may have affected your relationship with food. If you are planning to see a therapist as apart of your journey. Set a goal date for this. Do the research and write it in the notes of this chapter. And take action - make the appointment.

_____

_____

_____

_____

_____

_____

_____

4.

Raise the standard

WHILE INHALING THE smell of brand new carpet, the fresh paint and seeing the shinny new equipment; my immediate thought was... do I belong here? Is this really for me to partake of?

This was the thought I had after joining a gym that was in my new neighborhood which was far more affluent than what I was exposed to growing up. I nervously and cautiously joined the gym that day; because I knew I needed to shed some pounds and because I quickly noticed how everyone in the area was so active. They were either in the gyms, biking, skating or were participating in triathlons. I was really attracted to the women's running groups I saw running through the streets in perfectly cool October weather.

I saw families working out together or the kids were at football practice, soccer practice or whichever sport was in season at the time.

And I wanted it! I wanted to join this life style of movement! I wanted to breathe in this clean fresh air and admire the palm trees as I drove in the neighborhood. Although my family's income said I belonged there... my head didn't fully believe it.

Growing up - I could only recall the dingy boys and girls club in my neighborhood that was often painted caution light yellow or a deep depressing purple on alternating years. We also had a local park in the back of our neighborhood that I could never go to because of the sketchy behavior that took place there.

As I began to participate in the group activities, hire a trainer and workout next to what seemed to be the most athletic people I had seen outside of television… I began to talk to myself internally.

Yes… you do belong here, this is for you, and you will succeed here.

See, what I needed to do was raise my level of expectation. I needed to **raise my standard**.

I needed to tell myself that not only did I belong there… I should except nothing less.

I deserved to workout in a nice gym, meet new people and improve my level of physical activity.

Raising The Standard - is a personal rule or expectation about the level of excellence we require in something.

Whether we realize it or not; we all have personal standards that determine the quality of work we do, our personal hygiene, how we treat people and even our punctuality - are we always late or on time?

We have standards regarding the type of clothing we wear, the kind of car we drive, how often we get our hair done and get that manicure. For the most part the decisions we make early in life about what we can have or what we can do are based upon how we were raised or our general environment.

But can we change the standard? Can we expect more? Can we have or experience more?

Sure we can!

So why don't we have that same thought process - when it comes to our health?… many of us have just been stuck; and have just settled with the way things are.

Stop Settling for the norm-

We go year after year being overweight because we have set the standard that being overweight is OK, even if we're not happy about it. We have set the standard that just plopping on the couch every evening is OK. We have set the standard the our hairstyles are more important than being active and getting a little sweaty.

We have set the standard that others come before us and we struggle with making self-care a priority.

Laura's expression about self-care:

I have struggled with my weight most of my life because self-care was not a priority. I poured all of my energy into providing for my family, building a career and trying to make life as colorful as possible. I associated self-care with selfishness. Why? I do not know. It was the lowest of my priorities. I thought my source of happiness and self-worth was defined by how much of myself I gave to others, not knowing that I was really just wearing myself out. I was always taught to esteem others (family, the church, friends) before myself and I think a lot of women, including myself, believe this somehow translates to sacrifice of self.

I was having issues with high blood pressure after several appointments and I did not want to be on medication or worst, die. So, I made a decision that I wanted to live my best life and a commitment to myself to stop putting myself last. Honestly, I just changed my mind. They say a changed mind is a powerful thing and it really is. I changed the way that I perceived self-care. Instead of feeling like I had to choose between taking care of myself and others, I told myself that I could not

be a blessing to anyone if I am dead. I changed the way that I viewed exercise. It was no longer my enemy but my new best friend. I woke up every morning ready to put in some work.

I got real with myself. I shifted my perception of self-care from self-centeredness into self-preservation and it has been one of the greatest gifts that I could have ever given myself.

I have lost some weight along the way (22lbs and counting), but I have gained so much more than I have lost. I found my strength, my peace, and my balance.

We have to tell ourselves that our old standards are no longer working and its time to raise them!

Believing I could-

See regarding my gym experience - I didn't believe in my head that I belonged in a gym that nice and to be mingling among the athletic elite. Although my environment had changed, my thinking... my perspective had not.

I needed to start believing I deserved to be there. I needed to change my personal requirement about how and where I worked out for exercise. **I needed to require my internal level of excellence to match what I saw visually on the outside.**

Mentally it was tough to do for a while because I couldn't help but think of how in the urban community I was from; you just didn't see people jogging or biking outside. It was more like seeing guys hanging out on the corner. So if you were serious about working out you had to find a gym or park where you felt more safe.

36

As I adapted to my new area, I had to Raise the Standard in several ways and I want to encourage you to do the same regardless to where you live geographically and what your income is.

"We all act consistent with who we believe we are"
Tony Robbins

Dining Like A Queen-

Another way of raising my standard was my food choices. I made the switch from the greasy chicken in the box and prepackaged foods; to protein enriched foods, complex carbohydrates, fresh green vegetables and healthy fats.

If I was going to be successful at dropping the weight, I had to require a better quality food. No one else was doing the grocery shopping for me; so the I had to make it mandatory that I was no longer going to buy certain foods. I had to make the switch from processed cold-cut meats and greasy potato chips because they were inexpensive and easy. I had to decide that eating from the dollar menu from those restaurant chains were no longer going to fit into my goal-set.

The struggle was real:

My greatest struggle with raising the standard was with what I put in my mouth! I had a serious sweet tooth and would always crave sweets on a daily basis. I would eat anything from doughnuts from the bakery to (2) packages of Little Debbie cakes; or an entire large bag of potato chips to satisfy the salt craving after eating the sweets.

Isn't it interesting how we crave sugar after eating salty things or vice versa? There is a scientific reason behind our cravings and we will discuss later.

This relationship I had with junk food took my blood pressure to extremely high levels. When I ate that way before bed, I would take a couple of baby aspirin in hope to keep my heart from the fast palpitations because of my rising blood pressure.

My eating habits were just a wreck and out of control!

The Decision-

I want you to know today that you really can eat healthier food and afford it. It has been proven that we can get a quick fast-food meal at a cheaper cost than healthier food choices at our local grocer. But if you are going to raise the standard and require better for yourself and your family; you may need to re-evaluate what you are spending your money on and just decide to adjust and make it work.

For example, If you have a family of four and decide to go to the local drive thru; you are probably going to spend at least twenty five -dollars. Maybe even more. Ask yourself… can I take that same $25 and buy a family pack of chicken (and grill or bake it), veggies and maybe some red potatoes to make a meal at home? Sure you can! And probably have leftovers for mom and dad to take for lunch the next day.

Decide you are going to invest the time into locating affordable grocers where you can purchase better quality food vs the fast quick solution.

I often visit a local butcher where they process and cut the meat in house and the meat is of good quality, really fresh and affordable. The shop has been in existence since I was a child and they have always been a go to spot for me. The drive for me now to the butcher is at least 25 miles but its worth the investment for the quality of product and the savings vs eating out often.

Needless to say - if you plan, budget and execute the plan; you can enjoy steak, shrimp and quality cuts of meat if you make the choice to. What are you willing to give up? Where else can you scale back in your finances to ensure that you and the family are making healthier food choices that aid in your weight loss journey?

If budget is not an issue...

For many of us... finances are not the issue. We eat the way we do because we have become addicted to high calorie - carb rich foods and it has just become the norm for us and our family members just follow suit.

Do it no matter what...

Lets' say you have personally committed to eating better and your family isn't ready to change. Don't settle for the greasy foods that are drenched in transfats... it's time you raise your own standard. Raise your personal standard by cooking a separate healthier meal just for you. If you're waiting on your spouse or best friend at lunch to make better food choices with you and they aren't interested; it's time to raise your standard and go it alone.

There were plenty of times when I skipped dessert or refused to eat sweets late at night with my husband because I had a goal in mind. You will have family and friends that say... "its Okay in moderation." And yes its true... having dessert is Okay within moderation... but let's be honest - everyone's version of moderation is different.

So raising the standard is a very personal thing... your standard may be different from your spouse's standard although you have a lot in common and share many beliefs.

The standards you set about your health - the food you eat - the way you choose to exercise - has to be an individual walk for you.

Increasing in knowledge-

Another area I needed to raise my standards was in the area of self-education! I needed more information. The myths and assumptions I took for gospel truth regarding improving my health were wrong. The things I tried and thought were right... simply were not sustainable.

I was in search of the proper information to insure I would finally change my health for good. I had to log out of one social media site because I was spending too much time just watching other people's lives! I began to focus and follow sites or videos that were going to help me expand my knowledge base about improving my health. Most importantly, I was in search of nutritional knowledge and to become more aware of food & practices that contributed to disease.

I had a determination that I was going to eat, breathe, sleep and even dream of weight loss. I was going to read about it, listen to broadcast about it until it was downloaded into the very core of me! I was determined to have tunnel vision about living a healthier life until it became a reality for me.

I was able to find a few people that really knew their stuff about diet and exercise. The people I gave my attention to were a few personal trainers and a couple of health & wellness coaches.

Day after day, I listened closely and took notes while working at my desk or cleaning the house.

New Environments - New Experiences

As you raise your standard in the areas of what you eat, when you eat and making the choice to become more active; I want to encourage you to have balance in this process.

Raise the standard in your level of play - If you have been mentally living in a box and your routine has become redundant; I want you to give yourself permission to try new places, new experiences and be open to meeting new people. Go back to the hobbies or crafts you used to enjoy as you move through your weight loss journey. The days of feeling guilty for doing something you enjoy, something just for you are over! We only get one body, one life and its imperative that we balance hard work and discipline with fun and enjoyment in our lives.

I can recall going out with a work - out buddy that I met at the gym. We had different belief systems when it came to certain things but we would often dine together, shop together and our kids would play together. I learned things from her and she learned things from me.

As you progress through this journey - make the commitment that you will indeed try new things and experience new places while you are in this transition. It just makes us happier people!

Action Required 1:

In the space provided below answer the following questions:

What does raising the standard look like for you personally?

_____

_____

_____

_____

_____

Identify which area(s) you need to raise your standard. Could it be your food selections, being more active, your environment, or adding more play to your journey?

_____

_____

_____

_____

_____

Action Required 2:

Write an apology letter to yourself; apologizing for the mistreatment to your body. Grab a separate sheet of paper if necessary.

Apologize to your body if you have taken it for granted or even abused it over the years. Tell your one and only body how you will treat it moving forward.

_____

_____

_____

_____

_____

_____

_____

_____

_____

_____

5.

Getting Started

I WAS SICK OF myself! I had - had enough! I was in miserable pain and had been up all night. I literally had a stomach ache from overeating throughout the day and I couldn't sleep at all.

It pained me to sit still in one place and it was painful to lie in bed. I paced the floor the entire night and drank warm water with baking soda in hope to bringing myself some relief. The pain was so bad that I actually cried and I was in mental anguish because I was angry with myself for overeating again!

Since the warm carbonated water didn't bring any relief; I knew the only thing that would was going to help me was - time. I had to give my digestive system time to realign. I felt so bad, I couldn't eat anything the next morning if I wanted to! I also missed work the next day. By 5 or 6 am - I felt some relief but I was too sleepy and exhausted from being up all night to work that day. I vowed to myself that morning that I would not eat again until I felt empty and just starving.

As the day progressed, I honored that vow and did not eat for another 12 hour or so. When I did decide to finally eat, I chose something light - it was actually soup broth because I did not want to over tax my stomach again and fall back into that miserable feeling that kept me up the night before.

After sipping on the broth my only meal that day was a simple salad; and I ate it several hours before bed time.

The switch flipped

The following day I decided to follow the same eating path. Upon waking I waited some where between 8 and 10 hours before I had my first meal. My food choices that day were on the lighter side just as the day before. In the midst of eating my salad that evening; it was as if a light switch turned on in my head! I was fasting! I had been practicing intermittent fasting for the past 2 days without realizing it. Of course, I had heard of it before and recall trying it several years prior with a friend.

But up until that moment... I had dismissed it; forgotten about it.

My next thought was... can I continue doing this? I was feeling better by delaying the time that I had my first meal and I slept good the second night because I had eaten much earlier before going to bed.

Over the next couple of days, I began to research intermittent fasting. I was interested and intrigued and really wanted to know what it was all about and how it worked.

See growing up, I was only really familiar with the word **FASTING** from my father and the church we attended. I was taught that fasting was for spiritual reasons only. We understood it as a way to cleanse your spirit so you could become closer to God. Fasting was actually not something we enjoyed as children and young adults growing up in our church. It just seemed to be a hard task and if you committed to it in front of others - It just became a legalistic -rule driven process (at least in my mind).

But the more I looked into intermittent fasting to improve my health; the more I realized this was doable and it was for me.

See my initial approach with this was not to necessarily lose weight... but it was to feel better. I was tired of feeling crappy, bloated and fighting the acid reflux every night. The simplest thing eaten before bed seem to give me heart burn and make me belch all night. It was worse if I consumed something sugary before bed. I would actually be awakened by the feeling of my food coming up through my nose! I know... gross right?

So I made the decision that day that I was going to follow the path of intermittent fasting. I wasn't sure where it would lead me exactly; but I was on a mission to feel better in my body. I wanted to have more good nights of sleep. At this point in my life I also felt like I was my doctor's guinea pig.

We could not seem to get my blood pressure lowered to normal levels; so she was trying a different dosage of a particular medicine each month. I really disliked this process! See although my weight fluctuated over the years; I had never been prescribed medication by a doctor for high blood pressure until this point in my life. Had I been walking around with high blood pressure prior to seeing this doctor?

Yes!; sure - Because I could feel my heart palpating fast after I would eat a high caloric meal. I would also check my blood pressure at home from time to time. However, I was sort of self-treating myself when taking the baby aspirin daily or mainly at night because I knew that's what doctors gave heart patients to prevent heart attack or stroke.

Upon making this new decision to explore intermittent fasting; I also knew this was the last straw for me! This was the last battle I was going to fight with my weight. And I came in with guns blazing! This was a battle I was going to win!

Being that I had been on this roller coaster of good health habits and bad ones several times over the years... I knew that I needed some tools if I was going to succeed. I was tired of falling flat on my face after trying something for two or three months and giving up.

I began to think about the practices and behaviors that worked for me in the past and which didn't. After much thought, I knew that I needed: **Education** (about fasting), **Accountability** and I knew I had to be **Active** if I was going to win.

As mentioned, the majority of my experience in past years with fasting was for spiritual reasons. After deciding to fast for weight loss, I became hungry for knowledge about fasting. Any time that we are walking into new experiences that can be life altering; we must **Educate** ourselves on the topic. Before searching for help in the accountability area and getting active; I wanted to know of the different types of fast I could explore. I wanted to learn of the benefits of fasting and I also wanted to know if fasting had any down - sides or side effects. I wanted to explore what type of fast would work for me.

So I searched on -line, I purchased books and even asked total strangers questions about fasting. In my many years of living, I have noticed that many of us can have a tendency to jump right into things (especially weight loss journeys) without educating our selves. We try this or that, or give it very little effort and then give up… complaining… "it didn't work".

I wanted to know the science behind it. I read books by medical doctors on fasting. I read books and articles from common everyday people that decided to write about it after being successful at it for many years. I really wanted to know if I could fast for many hours without feeling like I was going to faint. I wanted to know if I could work for my clients and still keep up my normal day to day activity during those 8 or 9 hours and survive. Was I going to have headaches? Was fasting going to affect my blood pressure issue in a negative way and send me to the emergency room was my most pressing question.

See fasting for weight loss; was just far from the normal teaching about dieting I had received in years prior. We were taught to eat the 5 to 6 smalls meals per day to keep our metabolism going; which would result in weight loss.

I didn't want to just blindly walk into this. I was sick and tired of over-eating because I was bored, frustrated or stressed. I was sick of belly aches as a woman in her forties and walking around with a bloated belly and breast. Yep!... that's where the weight just sat on me.

I was looking for real results and decided to have the patience to get through the process.

Getting Help - Accountability

The greatest benefit of joining the weight loss programs and meeting weekly years prior was that it made me accountable to someone. When I was faithful with showing up; I saw results. When I would grocery shop or even dine out, I was conscious of what I bought and chose as a meal because I knew it would affect the scale. I wanted so bad each week for that scale to say that I had dropped a pound or two. I would stand on the large scale in front of those little old ladies and just hope they had good news for me. And when they didn't, they always had an encouraging comment.

When I went to group discussions, I would fully engage and get involved. I would discuss my struggles and victories. I participated in the (healthy) potlucks and community activity days. I was even asked to be a speaker and share my story at one of the events. The group gave me strength. It felt like a sense of community, a sense of togetherness. The check in every week was a good thing for me because I felt like I was not only doing it for me but for someone else too.

So as I began this remarkable journey of intermittent fasting; and after I had learned enough to at least get started; I knew I needed that sense of community. So I searched for it. Thanks to the World Wide Web - you can find just about everything online. I didn't have to look for a physical group that I could connect with. It took a matter of a few minutes through my social media page to find a fasting group. In fact, I joined about 3 or 4 as my interest in this fasting thing was peaked! It was like I had the support of 30,000 people! In these online groups you are able to ask questions and no one makes you feel stupid for asking. You can discuss your struggles or maybe a symptom you're having and there is a guaranteed that someone in the group has experienced the same issue and has a resolution for you. The greatest thing by connecting with online support… is that you have support at your fingertips and its free!

So I was OK with connecting with total strangers all over the country - and even in other countries to get support I needed. I took my focus off of things and people that were wasting my time. If I had any leisure time between work any of my other responsibilities… I was logging in to my helpful place. I was receiving encouragement and giving encouragement to other women that had the same problem as me.

See- when we can admit that we are over-eaters and realize that we can't go it alone, there is help available...we just have to reach out.

Over the years I have often mentally compared my overeating and constant up-hill-down-hill progress with my son's drug addiction. Addiction - regardless to whatever it is we are addicted to; can be a hard thing to overcome.

When we're struggling; the support and the accountability is what assist us in the journey. Accountability is an essential tool we need if we are going to finally live a healthier life.

The other component I needed to succeed was to be **Active**. Although I was increasing in knowledge about fasting and had joined the online groups for support… I was dreading the exercise. After a month and a half of consistent fasting; I knew I needed to start exercising but I also knew I had to keep it simple yet consistent.

Easing in-

When starting a weight loss journey it's important to not to over extend yourself with exercise. If you haven't exercised in a while; it's not wise to jump into trying push-ups and planks when your only form of exercise prior to starting has been to walk to the mail box. Or from your car to the grocery store door. If you try to do too much when starting out; you may injure yourself or feel it's too difficult to keep up; therefore, you quit.

So starting out, I walked 3 to 4 evenings per week for 30 to 45 minutes. I didn't walk very fast. I just wanted to get moving. In years past I had become a runner. So some days during my walk I was tempted to run but resisted because I wanted to avoid injury. Prior to starting my fasting journey, I had been physically inactive for nine months. So I knew that just being consistent was good enough in the beginning.

Establishing a pattern of consistency in the early stages of your journey is vitally important. I want you to visualize - the component mentioned here of: **Education**, **Accountability** and physical **Activity** as your tool kit. I encourage you to etch this in your brain. Write it down if you have to. Post it on the bathroom mirror. Write it on a sticky note and post it in your car. Having a plan, a foundation that you can build upon is key. It's like your life raft when things get shaky or scary. You remember and follow the foundation that got you started.

This journey will be challenging. There will be days that you want to quit and decide its too hard; but I promise you that staying focused on your why and using the tools provided in this book will get you through the hard moments and rough patches.

While practicing these principles, I chose to be quiet about my fasting process. The word fasting is a negative word to many; and family and friends are quick to say you are starving yourself!

I believe I waited about two months before I fully shared with my husband that I was fasting. He would come home from work

and I would serve him as I normally would, but just tell him I had already eaten (which was true). Or sometimes, I would move my eating window to the time frame that he ate dinner so we were eating together. Although my husband eventually became aware that I was fasting; and he was noticing my results in the early months; I still chose to keep it from extended family and friends until I had made significant progress. I also decided not to discuss or post progress pictures of myself on line to family or friends. But I did feel free to post them in my fasting safe place. Which were my social media fasting groups because I knew the information could not be shared outside of the group.

I even went to lunch with friends and they didn't know that the meal I was eating with them was my first meal in 20 hours. I did more eating than talking during these gatherings but they had no clue, that I was eating a plate full of seafood, veggies and a dinner roll; while still reversing my chronic health challenges at the same time!

I just didn't want anyone's opinion or negative comments about fasting to derail or discourage me.

Now let's make this personal for you. Are you ready to start with your tool kit? The decision is totally up to you - if you will let the world know of your journey or keep your news between you and close family or friends. If you decide to share with others that you are fasting, be sure it is shared with those you know will support you. In the coming chapters I will guide you and explain fasting in great detail as well as stepping up the exercise to be sure you see results.

Participation time:

In the space provided below

Write down your plan.

How will you implement Education, Accountability and Activity into your life on a daily basis?

_____

_____

_____

_____

_____

_____

_____

6.

Fasting-the game changer

FASTING? YOU MEAN - you go without food for how many hours? If that's how you lost the weight - I don't know about that! Girl you're crazy! These are just a few of the phrases or statements I would hear from family or friends that inquire about my weight loss. On a serious note: **Fasting has been the way to crush the constant craving** for junk food and the overall poor food choices I was making. So if you're still reading this book, it tells me you're interested in doing the work to meet your personal goals. It tells me you're ready for true change and tired of the cycle of losing and gaining the weight over and over again.

Hopefully while working through the previous units, you have to been able to identify your Why. I pray you have begun to raise the standard when it comes to your health; and been able to start healing from what or who may have been preventing your weight loss.

The horrible belly ache that I mentioned earlier is what caused me to stumble upon fasting and I have never looked back since that day. After many years of failed weight loss attempts; fasting was the game changer for me. And after reading and researching of how to start, I did just that. I decided I was going to pursue fasting for weight loss and I just wanted to live a better quality of life - health wise. I was just tired of overeating and feeling bad on a regular basis.

So lets jump right in and explain what fasting is so as you embark on this journey, you're informed and equipped to get started.

Fasting is in fact a broad and expansive subject and there are so many avenues an author can venture into when discussing fasting. However, my goal is to thoroughly explain the basics of fasting; in the simplest way possible so you have a good grip on how it works and to help you identify which type and method of fasting best suits you.

First, lets clarify **what fasting is Not**: Fasting is not a diet. A diet can be considered a special course of food to which a person restricts themselves, either to lose weight or for medical reasons. Also, diets are usually temporary because restricting yourself of certain foods can become unbearable and usually causes us to revert back to our prior food choices and behaviors. Secondly, and contrary to what friends and family will tell you; fasting is not starvation; hence - starvation is actually long-term and when someone is in starvation its because they don't know when and where their next meal is coming from. When you're choosing to fast, you have access to food and can stop fasting any time you want to refeed.

So what is Fasting? simply - put - its a timed approach to eating. Its deciding your cut off window to stop eating completely for a certain period of time. Its like a hard reset on your body. Just mentally visualize performing a hard reset on your cell phone or laptop if it has been giving you problems or not operating to its full potential. Fasting is just that for our bodies. In general a fast usually last from 12 to 24 hours. This may initially seem like a long time to go without eating, but I'm about 99 % sure you have done this before if you have ever had to follow a Doctor's orders by going to have blood drawn for laboratory results. Remember when - you were instructed not to eat or drink anything for at least

12 hours before your blood test? That was a fast! The purpose of fasting before having your blood drawn is so your test results are accurate. The minerals, vitamins, carbohydrates, fats and proteins that make up all the food and beverages we consume can impact blood level readings which is why we are asked to fast before going for lab test.

So... fasting by choosing to refrain from eating for a certain period of time; you will actually find to be a positive, freeing and even cost efficient experience. Especially as you learn how to tweak which time frames and methods of fasting work best for you.

If you have already mentioned to family or friends that you are considering fasting for weight loss, I'm sure you've heard many negative remarks or responses to your decision. I know... they are telling you that you're being too extreme and are afraid you're going to hurt yourself. Believe it or not fasting has been in practice for thousands of years and is one of the oldest therapies in medicine. Many of the great doctors of ancient times recommended it as an important part of healing and prevention. For instance, Hippocrates (the father of Western medicine) believed that fasting enabled the body to heal itself. In ancient cultures fasting was often demanded before going to war and for some it was a part of a coming-of-age ritual. Fasting has also played a key role in some of the world's major religions. For instance, the religion of Judaism has several fast each year. Another is in the region of Islam, where Muslims fast during Ramadam (the holy month); while Roman Catholics and Eastern orthodoxy fast for 40 days during Lent. Additionally in Christianity, Christ fasted for 40 days in the desert.

So if fasting has been done for hundreds and hundreds of years, we can most certainty do it today to improve our overall health including weight loss. In fact, its even easier to do today because there are so many resources and aids to help educate and motivate us; as well as inspiring examples from others to help us accomplish our goals.

Is Fasting Safe? - Who Should Fast?

Fasting for weight loss is intended for those individuals wanting to detoxify and eliminate the body of toxins and to give the internal systems a rest from insulin spikes every time food is consumed. Its for those wanting to improve their health and help modify the risk factors like diabetes and cardiovascular disease. Its also sought after by those wanting to lower cholesterol and blood sugar levels and for many other reasons that we will discuss in detail later.

When is it not safe? - Who Should Not Fast?

As mentioned in the disclaimer at the beginning of this book, it is best to consult your physician before starting or changing your dietary regimen to be sure fasting is safe for you to do.

However, fasting is is not recommended by health professionals for:

- Children under 18 years of age
- Pregnant women
- Breastfeeding women
- Individuals who suffer from anorexia or other eating disorders

Other areas of precaution - Individuals experiencing:

Gout, Type 1 or Type 2 Diabetes, Gastroesophageal Reflux (GERD) disease and individuals that are on medications. If you fall into any of these categories, I urge you to seek the advice of your health care professional before beginning. However, we will discuss how diabetics can fast later in this chapter as there are many with type II diabetes that have been successful with fasting.

What to know before starting - essential requirements-

Before beginning your fast, I'd like to point out some things to be sure your journey is a healthy and a successful one.

If you're serious about this new lifestyle of fasting you need to be willing to demonstrate certain quality of life habits or practices. These habits would include **getting enough sleep, getting enough fresh air; and drinking adequate amounts of water**. I know these may seem very simplistic but there are so many people in the world that don't see these components as important and are slaves to the rat race and busyness of daily living. Its really important that we are getting enough rest. Our bodies need at least 7 to 8 hours of sleep nightly; and good rest is essential as the body heals itself in several ways as we sleep. In fact after a couple of consistent months of fasting, you will find that you sleep much better and are able to experience a deeper sleep once your body has been acclimated to fasting. I began to notice my sleep pattern changing about a month and a half to two months into fasting.

Aside from the heart burn and acid reflux disappearing, I noticed that I was able to fall into a deep sleep and even dream very vividly once I started fasting. I literally felt like I was sleeping like a baby with no care in the world! I would wake up feeling fully rested and it was just a feeling I had never experienced before. This is because Intermittent fasting (which is the method I chose) can help build a stronger circadian rhythm, which helps us sleep deeper and better. A circadian rhythm is a natural, internal process that regulates the sleep-wake cycle and repeats on each rotation of the Earth roughly every 24 hours. Consistent eating patterns during our feeding window helps the body to adopt a consistent sleep schedule at night. Studies have even found that fasting may even reduce your night time awakenings and decrease leg movements. In my research, it was surprising to find there is actually a scientific reason as to why and how we are able to get better sleep from fasting!

Don't skip the H2O - There are many reasons why our bodies need water and if you're one that usually skips it, I'd like you to see it as an essential component to your fasting and weight loss success. We need water to digest our food and to help remove waste from our bodies. Its needed help us pee and poop - you know it gets the digestive system on track. Another important reason why we need water is that is necessary for each cell in our bodies to work.

Get some sun!

Believe it or not; Adequate sunlight, yes!... getting outside - is essential while fasting as well. Just as fasting can eliminate unwanted toxins from our bodies, this is also achieved when we get out in the sun. Being exposed to adequate sun helps improve the blood circulation in the body. Also when we are exposed to sunlight, our bodies produce Vitamin D. Vitamin D helps us maintain calcium to prevent brittle, thin bones. So be willing to incorporate these healthy behaviors along with your fasting. The days of only getting 3-4 hours of sleep should be over for you and the complaint of "I don't like water" should be a statement of the past. You will find that the more you drink water, the more your body will crave it. Before you know it, picking up that water bottle will become second nature to you.

What happens in our bodies when we fast?

First off, when we eat, we absorb more food energy that we can immediately use; so some of this energy needs to be put away for use later. The primary hormone involved in both the storage and use of food energy is **insulin**. As a result, insulin rises when we eat our meals. When we consume proteins and carbohydrates (which are macronutrients) during our meals they both stimulate insulin. For those of us that have experienced high blood pressure, remember when you would eat the bread or the doughnut and very soon after, you felt uncomfortable, or may have even felt a little ill or maybe even light headed? This is because our insulin levels are increased after consuming those refined carbohydrates. The same goes for when we consume protein. Now this does not mean that we won't ever eat carbohydrates or proteins anymore but we will discuss in the next chapter some healthy carbohydrates and proteins that will not have our insulin levels all over the place when do eat them in our feeding window. Then there is fat, the third component of macronutrients - when we consume it believe it or not, it triggers a smaller amount of insulin because we rarely eat fat alone. Think about it - how many of you have just sat and ate a teaspoonful of oil or butter all by itself? Probably none of us right?

Its important to discuss what happens when we eat so we have a good understanding of what takes place in the body when we fast. As classically described by Jason Fung, MD: Insulin has two important functions. One is that it allows the body to immediately start using food energy. The second job of insulin, is that it helps store the excess energy. An example of this would be if you ate a large meal and your body didn't need that much glucose right away, insulin helps the body to store it and convert to energy later. This happens by turning the extra food into larger packages of glucose called glycogen, as a result glycogen is stored in the liver and muscles.

Fasting - Mode On

The process just described above - of using and storing food energy is reversed or is the opposite when we are in our fasting window. Our insulin levels drop, notifying the body... to start burning stored energy. The glucose that is housed in the liver is the most easily accessible energy source; as a result the liver stores enough to provide energy for 24 hours or so. After that time frame the body then starts to breakdown stored body fat for energy. To simplify this, the body really only exist in 2 states - the feeding (high insulin) and the fasted (low insulin) state.

See we are either storing food energy or we are burning it. **The process of the body burning the stored fat is what results in weight loss for us.** See- what I never knew before fasting is that being in the constant state of eating - even if it was healthy food; wasn't producing the weight loss results I was looking for because my insulin was constantly working.

Why Fasting works vs traditional dieting-

For at least the past 20 to 25 years, we have been taught to eat 5 to 6 small meals a day to keep our metabolism going. We were even taught to count every single calorie and log the food we consumed. We've been told that the only way to lose weight is by the calories in - calories out method - you know to eat fewer calories than you expend. It has also been explained that the excessive caloric intake is what causes us to be obese (which is partially true). The general consensus from medical professionals and trainers when we didn't achieve our goals from counting and recording; was... it's our fault that we are still overweight because we haven't been putting in enough effort.

According to Dr. Fung (medical doctor and author of the obesity code): The underlying cause of obesity is actually a hormonal imbalance vs a caloric imbalance. What we have to understand here is that insulin is a fat storing hormone and the more frequent we are eating throughout the day (spiking the insulin levels) - is why we aren't losing the weight and remaining obese.

To be honest, as I began to research this fasting thing... this was hard for me to swallow. It was hard for me to believe because we've been taught by medical professionals and fitness trainers the exact opposite of fasting. And if we would take a moment by doing some self-inventory; and be honest with ourselves - eating several small meals throughout the day just hasn't worked!

Friends, I can honestly say that fasting has been by far the easiest, healthiest and most sustainable way I have been able to lose the weight and keep it off; and there is no turning back!

Calories - To count or not to count?

Yes, It's been etched in our brains over the years to check labels for sodium, sugar and carbohydrate percentages; as well as the number of calories we're taking in. While it is still vitally important that we monitor how much sodium, sugar and carbohydrates we are eating, we can't necessarily see counting calories as "The gospel truth" like we've been made to think before.

Here's why: turns out, counting calories is not an exact science and is fundamentally flawed. In a publication by Dr.'s John Berardi and Helen Kollias; the doctors confirm: - the principles of energy balance do work - meaning if we take in more calories/ energy than we expend, we gain weight. Take in fewer calories/energy than we expend, we lose weight.

However, counting calories to control your energy intake is not necessarily true. There are several reasons for this as explained in the publication: calorie counts are imprecise, we don't absorb all the calories we consume, the way food is prepared changes its calorie load, individuals absorb calories uniquely and variably and; lastly because we aren't great at eyeballing portion sizes. I'm sure like me, you can recall putting a little bit of food on the plate and trying to gauge or guess how many calories the portion was - and sometimes if we felt it was too little, we would add on another spoonful or two. You know a little more won't hurt. This is why counting calories isn't always as accurate as we think and personally I am glad I'm no longer a slave to calorie counting.

So Let's dive into Fasting in more detail:

Types of Fast-

Now that we understand how fasting works and how it affects our bodies, I'd like to discuss in detail the 4 different types of fasting. I found in my journey that trying different fasting methods was good just for the experience of change and most importantly when I experienced a stall in my weight loss, changing the type and method of how I fasted was a key factor is breaking the stalled progress.

Intermittent Fasting-

So what's all they hype? We all hear the term so much... Do we believe the hype? Does it work? & What is it exactly?

Intermittent fasting is simply a pattern - It's a pattern where you cycle between periods of eating and fasting. The length of a person's fasting and feeding window can vary widely. We can choose to fast from 12 hours for up to several days at a time. There are many variations of intermittent fasting and one regimen may work for one person but not be as effective for another. So it really all boils down to personal choice. However, I'd like to keep things simple and straight forward and explain different intermittent fasting schedules and I encourage you to start small and simple but be willing to change things up so you get to experience the different schedules. This is encouraged also because we all have different life and work schedules. For instance, someone that works a 9-5 job may need a different fasting schedule from someone that may work an overnight job. I also encourage you to try the different variations of intermittent fasting because you will notice some positive changes in your body and overall health as you dig deeper into longer fasting periods. You will find that there is power (better results) in longer fasting periods.

For beginners or newbies to fasting, it is recommended that you start with a 12 or 16 hour fast.

12-hour fasting is considered a short daily fast and would be a great start for newbies to establish a pattern of consistency or to sort of stick your toe in the water. An example of 12 hour fasting would be to have a feeding window from 7am to 7pm. If your habits have been to eat or snack late at night - followed by going to bed shortly after; this has probably contributed to your weight gain over the years. A 12 hour fast would be a great way to introduce fasting so it doesn't seem so daunting or extreme in the beginning.

In earlier years, a twelve-hour fasting period was normal and most people would eat their three meals a day within the twelve-hour window. This was pretty standard with American dieters until the late 1970's. This is when we started to adapt to a higher carbohydrate, lower-fat diet. These changes began with the publication of the USDA's Dietary Guidelines for Americans in 1977. This is significant because as discussed, diets high in refined carbohydrates stimulate high levels of insulin on a consistent basis. And as we know - high levels of insulin makes us gain weight and result in obesity and for some of us morbid obesity.

While 12 hour fasting is a good start you may find it not to be powerful or long enough to see some changes on the scale especially depending on what you are consuming with the three meals in that window. Longer fast are usually required to really see a difference. The concept is the same as when we start working out. Instead of jumping right into high intensity sprints; start by simply walking consistently for the first 30 days to establish a pattern of consistency.

16:8 Method is actually where I started and can actually be as simple as not eating anything after dinner and skipping breakfast. An example of this would look like finishing your last meal at 8pm and not eating until noon the next day. This would mean that technically you are fasting for 16 hours. This will take some getting used to if you have always been a breakfast eater. You know since we have been programmed to believe that breakfast is the most important meal of the day. The great thing about fasting and what I have personally found to be true is that its **"Flexible, Free and Fuels Fat loss"** So because it is **flexible** - you can change up the time frame for your 16/8 to what works best for you. Personally, 8:00pm for me was too late to eat my last meal since I'm usually in bed and asleep by 9pm. Regardless to what I chose to eat; an 8pm meal would have taken me back to the acid reflux issues.

When starting 16/8, I usually had my last meal at 6:45 or 7pm and would usually have my first meal at 11am the next day. And guess what? If I wanted breakfast-food at 11am - I would eat that. If I wanted lunch as my first meal I would eat that. Fasting can be **free** in a couple of manners - free in the literal sense of - you save money because you find you're not spending as much money on food as you did before. Let's face it - If you're not eating - you're not shopping for grocery or in the drive thru lines like before. I was always a breakfast person and had to have my coffee with breakfast. I mean I just felt like I was going to have a rough day or couldn't do my job effectively if my belly was not full from a chicken biscuit with strawberry jam, tater - tots and lemonade with light ice from my favorite restaurant. Its also offers **freedom** and **flexibility** in the sense of you deciding which 16 hour window works for you not to eat. As long as its 16 consecutive hours of no eating, you're good to go - and you're free to do what works for you. Fasting definitely **fuels fat loss** in the body; we start to see the numbers go down on the scale as a result of lower insulin levels because we're not constantly eating. The reverse to this is when we are eating too often throughout the day, our insulin levels are high thereby preventing the body from dropping the weight.

In general on this schedule, most people do skip their morning meal everyday. But the number of meals you choose to eat within your 8 hour window is totally up to you. Some choose to eat three meals within the 8 hours and some choose to eat two. This method for most people is fairly easy to incorporate into their daily lives because it means skipping breakfast and fitting lunch and dinner into an 8 hour window. I personally found that two meals were sufficient for me and I combined low carbohydrate dieting with my fasting. Aside from wanting to feel better, I wanted the weight off! I was sick of looking like a football player! I generally carried my weight in my upper body - I was just wide up top - large breast, broad shoulders, fat arms and bulging belly.

So as I adapted to this method, I would limit the amount and type of carbohydrates I would eat. On this regimen, you will find that weight loss tends to be slow but steady.

My dear friends; please... don't be discouraged by the word slow... remember... the goal is sustainability. What ever you do to lose the weight is what you have to keep doing to keep it off.

So I know the liquid weight loss potions being sold by your friends on social media are attractive and they are seeing quick results; but just watch them over the next several months to see if its sustainable. You can't take pills and potions for the rest of your life to stay slim. However, fasting is sustainable and can be a life long enjoyable experience to improve your quality of life. I know from personal experience, when we get tired of buying that stuff, we blow right back up and are quiet about it!

20 Hour Fast- is just as it sounds. It consists of fasting for twenty hours and only eating within a four- hour window. I often did this method without realizing it. If I got busy with work or a project, I would often extend my time from 16 to 20 hours. I know it may be hard to believe but there will be times that the longer you fast, you won't feel hungry and may have to make yourself eat. I would usually have a small snack when my eating window started and then my 1 larger meal a couple of hours later. I would also change this up by having my meal at the first start of the four- hour window and maybe a little dessert within the last hour to thirty minutes of the window. Either way - I would be sure and consume all that I was going to eat that day within the four- hour window and then begin the fasting cycle again.

Another version of 20 hour Intermittent fasting was generated by Ori Hofmekler in his 2002 book:

"The Warrior Diet". Hofmekler was actually a member of the Israeli Special Forces who transitioned into the field of fitness and nutrition. The warrior diet briefly explained is based upon the practices of ancient warriors such as the Romans and Spartans; in which they ate very little during the day and feasted at night. Hofmekler tweaked it to his own version in which one is to consume small amounts of dairy products, hard boiled eggs, raw fruits and vegetables, as well as fluids that are zero calories during the twenty-hour fasting period. After the fasting period, participants could essentially eat any foods they want within the four- hour window. Although the warrior diet fasting method has been a popular one over the last several years and many have benefited from it; I have to be honest and say I tried it for a couple of days but did not adopt it as a normal fasting method for myself. I felt it was fair to mention the warrior diet to offer you another variation of fasting. You may try it and find that it works great for you.

As for me- sometimes I can be an" all or nothing type of girl". I saw better results with not eating at all within the twenty-hour window and consuming all of my daily food within the four- hour time frame. However, some days I would keep it light and have raw veggies and fruit as a snack in my feeding window and maybe a large salad and steak as my dinner meal. As I mentioned earlier- fasting can and will produce fat loss. I saw great results on the scale as I learned and practiced fasting for twenty hours or more.

This leads me to discuss Extended Fasting Periods-

Before taking on fasting periods longer than twenty hours, I suggest mastering or at least becoming comfortable and consistent with the shorter fasting windows to be sure you are ready for longer fasting. We can set ourselves up for failure if we try to jump right into a 48 to 72-hour; or even longer fast just because we're excited and think we can handle it. Fasting in my opinion becomes a craft and an art for an individual and one definitely has to practice self discipline to do it. However... the discipline is developed gradually. The more you do it, the more consistent you are, the easier it becomes. It then becomes second nature. There is no question of what am I eating for breakfast in the morning? Because I simply don't eat in the morning. I enjoy a cup of coffee between 5 and 6am and my first meal is later in the day depending on which method of fasting I'm currently using. So starting with the basics as mentioned and being consistent with those basics will take you farther into the fasting journey and the process will be easier if you have worked your way up to prolonged fast.

Now that we are discussing prolonged fasting, I wanted to mention a benefit of increasing your fasting hours and this starts to occur in the body between hours 18 to 20 but really kicks in with maximal benefits when you reach 48 to 72-hours of fasting.

This process is called **Autophagy** - Autophagy is like a self-cleaning. Its the body's way of cleaning out damaged cells to rejuvenate newer ones.

If we take the word apart: "auto means self and "phagy means eat". So the literal definition of autophagy is: self-eating". I know this may sound a little disgusting that this is happening to your body as you fast but it's actually beneficial to your overall health.

Another explanation of autophagy is the process where cells degrade and recycle their components, it provides fuel for energy and building blocks for cell renewal.

Cells also use autophagy to get rid of of damaged proteins and organelles, to counteract the negative effects of aging in the body. So yes, the more we fast and reach autophagy, we look younger! Another point about the benefits of autophagy is that after we experience and infection in our bodies, autophagy can destroy bacteria and viruses.

Scientist say Autophagy was first discovered in the 1960's but became more notable by Yoshininori Oshumi a Japanese cell biologists in the 1990's. He also won the Nobel Peace prize in 2016 for his discoveries in autophagy.

Since I began fasting, I can definitely identify with how the state of autophagy gives ability to counteract the negative effects to aging. There was a drastic change with the appearance of my skin. My face really took on a more youthful look and was very noticeable within my 7th to 8th month of fasting.

Aside from my weight loss I would constantly hear from family and friends that I looked so much younger and they would often say I was aging backwards. I heard the term so much that one day I decided to compare my photos. I located one that I took 3 years ago at age 44 and it was a photo I had snapped with a friend after a workout. I also pulled a current photo at age 47 and I could not believe the difference! I really did look younger. The crow's feet around my eyes were gone and my skin tone was brighter and just younger. The scars and blemishes I had were gone as well. It was almost just unbelievable. I shared the photo with my fasting group online and a few even commented that the picture of me at 44 looked as if I was the older sister of the 47-year-old me.

The 24-hour fast-

Involves fasting from breakfast to breakfast, dinner to dinner or lunch to lunch. An example of this looks like finishing dinner at 6pm one evening and not eating until 6pm the next day. This is my personal favorite method of fasting is also known as **OMAD (one meal a day)**. Essentially it is the form of fasting that consist of 23 hours of fasting and having 1-hour of eating. While trying different fasting methods, I found this one to be most effective for me especially if I was exercising on a daily basis. I would usually eat on my lunch break at 2pm daily and eat my one meal between the time frame of 2pm to 3pm. This time frame worked best for me because

I usually went to a workout class at 6pm and having eaten 4 hours earlier did not make me feel sluggish or heavy while working out.

I would eat a variation of foods depending on what I had a taste for. I usually tried to stay within a low carb diet when doing OMAD but I also knew I needed to keep a balance. For instance,- I didn't always have salad or a plate full of veggies. When doing OMAD, while not necessarily having to count calories, I wanted to be sure I was eating enough food. Especially because my workouts at the gym were pretty intense.

A typical meal for me doing OMAD usually consisted of meat, veggies, fruit and sometimes a small dinner roll. If I was in the mood for dessert, I would skip the bread and have a cookie or a piece of cake. Remember, you can eat what you want in your feeding window regardless to which fasting method you choose; but I want to caution you if you are practicing 24-hour fasting to make sure that during your feeding window that you are con-suming adequate amounts of proteins, vitamins as well as min-erals by eating foods that are nutrient dense and unprocessed. So, gauging down on potato chips during your feeding window will not sustain you when you resume fasting.

When practicing OMAD fasting, be sure you eat until you are full (not stuffed) and you may want to consider focusing on low carb, high fat and unprocessed foods as much as possible (depending on your goals).

Again - it's about finding the balance; and girls if "Aunt Flo" has come to visit that particular week, you may find yourself desiring the piece of chocolate vs fruit.

I am often asked - What do you eat? We will dive more into this in the next chapter but my response is always - I eat real food! & I eat good!

A plate of grilled bourbon chicken breast, sautéed broccoli with caramelized onions and a couple of servings of fruit is delicious and sustains me longer than a prepackaged muffin or a bag of potato chips.

Let's face it - if you eat crappy while in your feeding window on a consistent basis; this will be a hard journey for you. Remember the "Crave"… the more we eat it, the more we desire it.

The choice

So, even with choosing a lifestyle of fasting; you have to ask yourself how bad do you want to see results? Thinking about the results you want to see helps you determine what you choose to eat in your feeding window. As I am writing this chapter, I am on vacation and currently thinking about what I am going to eat in my feeding window. And I can be totally honest and say that vacation time as well as celebrating the holidays will be challenging. Vacations put us in a relaxed state of mind and there are so many food choices and just extra stuff available at your fingertips that aren't stocked in our fridge and cupboards at home. I will definitely have coffee this morning and can pick it up from the hotel lobby.

As I walk to the coffee machines, there are tons of muffins, snack bars and pastries offered as a complimentary breakfast to the patrons. I have to remember my goals and by pass that stuff. Its even in my hotel room! Because my husband eats it… LOL! So, while enjoying my coffee, I can think about the meal I will enjoy today as a late lunch or early dinner. I already have the restaurant mapped out. I will have a surf and turf meal which will consist of a 6oz steak, lobster, steamed broccoli and my favorite- a crab cake. So, I want you to know that I have been and am still in the journey with you. Although I have met my goal weight; I have to continue to do the work to maintain it.

Additional Extended Fast:

36-72-hour fast

As you become more experienced with fasting, I encourage you to try longer fast. Sometimes, our bodies just need a good overall detoxing and a reset. One thing to note about prolonged fasting is that there may not be a huge amount of weight loss; or you can regain some of the pounds lost after you refeed; however prolonged fasting tends to heal things that are wrong with us. An example is that some in the fasting community report that their joint pain went away, or they saw a huge reduction in acne as well as skin tags disappearing.

Many that suffer from type II Diabetes have benefited from 36 hour fasting. According to Dr. Jason Fung in his IDM Program, they used 36 hour fasting three times per week with **diabetic patients** on a continual basis until desired results were achieved. The patients were able to go off of all diabetes medications and reached their desired weight loss goals. Now this process can take some time. It's not like you do a 36 or 48 hour fast 1 to 2 times and expect to be cured from type II diabetes. This length or amount of extended day fasting segments depends on how long or many years the patient has been suffering from diabetes.

Studies have shown that patients newly diagnosed with type II diabetes have seen great success with fasting to reduce their A1C levels. As mentioned, I urge you to seek the advice from your physician if you have been diagnosed with type II diabetes before you start fasting; and to also go for check up's often once you start fasting. Connecting with other diabetics in the online fasting communities also helps.

I also want to caution you to be sure you are drinking plenty of water and non-caloric liquids should you choose to embark on one of these longer fast. Personally, the longest extended fast I have done is a 72-hour fast. Surprisingly, I did not feel very hungry much during the 72-hour fast. There were times that I felt a little weak, but I had done some research prior to starting the extended fast so that I was equipped. I purchased bone broth in case I had to sip on it. I was prepared to drink a little cup of coffee if I experienced hunger pangs. But most of all I prepared an electrolyte drink that I sipped on throughout the 3 days of no food intake. I was able to rely on this and did not find it necessary to drink coffee, tea or bone broth to help me through. However, just know that everyone's experience maybe different. Many fast with only water and not an electrolyte concoction.

The electrolyte drink consisted of Pink Himalayan salt, turmeric, apple cider vinegar, water and lemon juice. This actually taste good to me!, and we don't have to reinvent the wheel here. I simply saw the recipe online but changed the measurements to my liking. I also purchased a beautiful cup with a cute little straw that made me feel good about carrying the cup everywhere I went that weekend. I kept my extended fasting a secret from my family because I did not want to hear any negativity. When it was time to break the fast, I honestly was not very hungry and did not have a hard time with the fast overall. I believe this was because I had already been used to at least doing 24-hour fast on a weekly basis.

However, I must warn you that you can experience gas and bloating while extended fasting. Something that helped me with the bloating was that I drank a few cups of hot water during the day for relief. I must also clarify that I did not just jump from fasting from 24 hours to doing a 72-hour fast. My first intentional extended fast was a 48 hour fast. So, we have to work our way upwards. I also felt very different after the longer fast. I just felt like I was really purifying or detoxing my body during the three days without food. The body most definitely taps into your fat reserves when fasting this long. Researchers have also found that we can reset our immune system with 72-hours of fasting.

Never in my 47 years of living would I had ever thought I could go without one drop of food for 3 days; but I made it! So don't shy away from prolonged fast because they initially seem daunting. Just work your way up to the process. You may also find the need to try an extended fast should you hit a plateau in your weight loss. Another reason I participate in 3 day fast is to simply reestablish my fasting discipline. Let's face it, this journey will not be a perfect one and sometimes you will get off track. So for me, when I notice my eating getting out of hand a little, I crush the crave with a 3 day fast.

The 5:2 Diet

Is a form of fasting developed by Dr. Michael Mosley a television producer and physician based in the UK and is the bestselling author of his book **The Fast Diet**.

The 5:2 diet consist of having 5 days of eating as you normally would and on the 2 fast days, it instructs women to consume 500 calories and for men 600 calories. The 2 fasting days can be done back-to-back or spaced out. For example you can choose to fast on Sunday and Monday and only consume 500 calories if you're a female and 600 calories if you're a male. On Tuesday through Saturday of that week you would resume to your normal way of eating. Again, I would caution you to remember your goals on your eating days should you embark on this form of fasting. The Fast diet in my opinion is good for beginners that are just starting to fast to get comfortable with the process. However- I think you will find that you are well capable of fasting without food; then you may initially think so. You've got this! I'm rooting for you!

Alternate Day Fasting (ADF)

Just as it sounds- ADF is just that. Its abstaining from food for 1 full day and resuming your normal pattern of eating the following day. There are actually two variations with this method. One is to totally fast from eating on the fasting day and the other is that you are allowed 500 calories on the fasting day. Many fasters use their own discretion with this method of fasting. There are many that report that consuming the 500 calories helps them to make it through and they don't feel so deprived while on the other hand some fasters report that they truly fast on the non-feeding day. Both methods have proven weight loss results from fasters. So, it comes down to personal preference.

ADF is a fasting method that I did personally try during my weight loss journey and I actually enjoyed the change up from my OMAD and 16/8 regimen. When I followed the ADF method I chose not to eat at all on the fasting day and just to drink my morning coffee and water throughout the day.

Liquid Fasting

Is a form of fasting where one only consumes water, juice or broth and its usually done for a 24-hour period. No food at all is consumed and the liquids consumed are clear. Liquid fasting is recommended only once per week and can be an alternative to your normal fasting schedule. Research on liquid fasting indicates it helps to improve the digestive system. Also, according to a study in the American Journal of Cardiology (A June 2012 publication); revealed that those that practice liquid fasting regularly showed a lower risk of heart disease and diabetes and often have a lower body mass index. Be sure and carefully approach liquid fasting with caution to be sure you are healthy enough to do a liquid fast and consult your physician to be sure its safe for you especially if you may be considering a liquid fast longer than 24 hours.

Fasters that have been in the game for a while and are more experienced with extended fasting will often venture into liquid fasting for much longer periods than 24 hours. Many may go as long as 3, to 7 days or more with only consuming liquids. The weight loss results from liquid fasting can vary from person to person especially depending on the types of juice and how often a person is consuming it. If the juice consumed contains sugar even if its natural, it can affect insulin levels and weight loss progress.

Another Variation of liquid fasting is Water Fasting -

Is simply fasting from food and water being the only source of liquid intake. When water fasting you also refrain from coffee, tea or any other beverages. While there is no set time frame for this type of fasting; it is generally suggested by physicians and fasting experts for a time frame of 24 hours to 3 days. Since the body is restricted of carbohydrates while water fasting, it uses fat in the body for the energy source thereby resulting in weight loss. I want to mention here that you will notice that many in the online fasting communities do water fasting for 20,30 and some even 40 days. Many report huge benefits from fasting that long and many drop some serious weight during the fast. Personally, I never found that necessary and usually stay within 3 days when I desire to prolong my fast.

Dry Fasting-

Is the most extreme form of fasting and its considered absolute fasting because it restricts food and liquid. Fasting experts only recommend it once every 3 to 6 months if you are healthy enough to dry fast. This form of fasting restricts water, broth, coffee and tea which is allowed in other forms of fasting. Dry fasting can be done with any of the fasting methods already discussed such as intermittent fasting for example. Fans of dry fasting attribute it to improved immune function, cell regeneration, reduced inflammation as well as skin benefits.

Individuals considering dry fasting are cautioned to consult with your physician before beginning and is definitely not recommended for beginners. Since the intake of water is prohibited, there is a high-risk of complications due to fasters being dehydrated. Personally, this method of fasting was not attractive to me because my daily water intake was always crucial to my overall well-being. Also, in my early days of fasting I was still striving to improving my blood pressure so for me daily water intake was necessary while fasting.

I have described the various forms of fasting to inform you as the reader of some different types of fasting so that you're aware of what is available as you navigate though your fasting journey. Who knows- you may find that liquid or dry fasting works for you and you maybe one that sees significant progress and benefits when trying these methods. But I implore you again to seek the advice of your physician especially if you are considering a liquid or dry fast.

Intermittent Fasting & (Keto) Ketogenic Diet

As I joined the online fasting community, I noticed many fasters in my group were also following the keto diet. The combining of keto and intermittent fasting is currently a hot trend in the health community today. Since we've already discussed what intermittent fasting is, I will give you a synopsis of keto dieting just in case you're not familiar with how it works. The ketogenic diet is a way of eating that consist of high fat intake and very low carb intake. Usually, the amount of carbohydrates allowed are 20 to 50 grams per day.

This low carb amount forces the body to rely on fats instead of glucose for its main energy source. Dieticians explain that in the metabolic process known as ketosis, the body breaks down fats to form substances called ketones that serve as an alternate fuel source. Following keto can be an effective way to lose weight and has several other benefits. Keto has been used for many years by physicians to treat epilepsy and shows promise for other neurological disorders. It reduces blood sugar, improves insulin resistance and lowers heart disease risk factors such as our triglyceride levels.

Many fasters that incorporate keto with intermittent fasting report that the fasting helps their bodies to reach ketosis quicker than just the keto diet alone. Why? This is because when fasting your body maintains its energy balance by shifting its fuel source from carbs to fats which is the exact premise of the keto diet. For those that struggle to reach ketosis while practicing the keto diet, adding intermittent fasting can be a great way to catapult your progress.

In my online fasting group, I would witness countless before and after pictures of women and men that had successfully lost significant amounts of weight from practicing both intermittent fasting and the keto diet. Combining the two is likely safe for most people however be sure and consult with your physician to be sure it is safe for you. Personally, I would incorporate keto with my fasting when I just felt like I needed a break from sugar intake. While I did not eat junk food often in my feeding window, sometimes I felt like a needed a break from the sugary fruit. I love fruit very much or maybe a glass of apple juice. I just knew from the scale and even internally when I needed to tone things back a bit to see better results. So, toning things back for me was to occasionally incorporate keto when in my feeding window. When practicing keto, I was able to eat blueberries, blackberries and strawberries vs the pineapples and grapes I love so much.

How Fasting Can Affect Our Hormones

There are many hormones in the body that are affected when we fast and I cannot conclude this chapter without discussing a few of them. I will focus on 4 endocrine hormones in particular to describe how fasting affects these hormones.

Insulin -Although this has been discussed earlier, I wanted to give a refresher on how insulin is affected in the body when we fast.

Insulin is a hormone that has several functions in the body's metabolism. It regulates how the body uses and stores glucose and fat. Also, many of the body's cells rely on insulin to take glucose from the blood for energy. In simple terms- insulin makes fat so the more insulin made, the more fat we store. So essentially when we are fasting, we give our bodies time to lower insulin levels, which reverses the fat storing process. As a result, when insulin levels drop, the process goes in reverse and we lose fat.

Human Growth Hormone(HGH) -

Is a small protein that is made by the pituitary gland and is released into the bloodstream. HGH production is controlled by a complex set of hormones produced in portion of the brain and in the intestinal tract and pancreas. The pituitary disperses bursts of growth hormone and our levels rise. Some examples of this would be when we see our newborn babies for the first time, when we fall in love, when we are hugged, following exercise, when we experience trauma and when we sleep. Scientists who carefully measure its production report that it's at its highest level when we are children, it peaks at puberty and declines from middle age and onward. As we age, HGH decreases in our bodies, we start to lose muscle mass and our skin starts to thin.

Cortisol -

Is considered a steroid hormone and is made in the cortex of adrenal glands and then released into the blood which transports it throughout the body. As our bodies perceive stress the adrenal glands make and release cortisol into the blood stream and this is often referred to as the stress hormone. When we are in stress mode and cortisol is released, we can see an increase in our heart rates and blood pressure. This is referred to as our natural "flight or fight" response that have kept us as humans alive for many -many years. If we are in constant high stress modes in our daily lives- this makes it difficult to lose weight. We may also suffer from bloating and fluid retention in our bodies because of the stimulation or constant release of cortisol in the body.

Something important to point out here is that fasting actually increases our cortisol levels especially when we are on extended fast. The body is stressed. This doesn't mean that we aren't to fast but knowing how to break your fast properly can lower our insulin and cortisol levels. A few examples of lowering the cortisol levels at the end of our fast would be to go for a walk if you can or take a nap just before ending the fast. If these are not possible, drink tea vs coffee when breaking your fast and cinnamon is a good source to use to lower cortisol levels when ending your fast.

Estrogen -
Is one of two main sex hormones that we have as women. The other hormone is progesterone. As we know, estrogen is responsible for our physical features as females as well as reproduction. Estrogen brings about physical changes that affect us from puberty to womanhood. It also helps control the menstrual cycle and is important for bearing our children. Some of its functions is to keep cholesterol in control, protect our bone health and it affects our brain (including our moods), heart, bones, skin and other tissues. For several reasons our bodies can make too little or too much estrogen. In addition our levels can change throughout the month. These levels are highest in the middle of our menstrual cycle and at their lowest during our periods. And for those of us that are in the forty plus club, we know estrogen levels drop as peri menopausal or post-menopausal women. **So how does fasting affect our estrogen?** While fasting is not recommended for females under 18, many women report correction and improvements in their menstrual cycle since adapting to a fasting lifestyle. Studies also report a dramatic improvement with women suffering from uterine fibroid tumors. When fasting properly many saw a reduction in size and effect of their tumors. Personally I have never suffered from fibroid tumors but I have definitely experienced a regulation of my menstrual cycle. Since fasting it shows up like clockwork for me and is

lighter in flow and less painful. I even notice a better mood during that time than I ever have before. Or to clarify, I feel less cranky and irritable.

Because we can still experience some hormone fluctuations during our cycle, getting in some exercise and eating foods that help balance our hormones is helpful. For example, consuming foods that boost serotonin can be helpful such as salmon, nuts , seeds, eggs, turkey or poultry and maybe even some pineapple. Serotonin is a mood enhancing chemical in the brain.

Great advise from the Doctor -

While my hormonal experience since starting to fast seems to be almost painless, many women have far more issues than I experienced. In my research I was enlightened by study from Dr. Mindy Pelz and began to put her advice into practice. The book she wrote concerning the information I will share is "The Menopause Reset". You can also find many of her fasting educational videos on YouTube.

Here's what I learned: and want to share it with you especially if you are one that has seen negative affects to your menstrual cycle since you started fasting.

*Women under 40 years old should not do extended or prolonged fasting during days 21-28 of your cycle. She explains this is because our bodies need to make progesterone. When we are doing prolonged fasting, our bodies are in ketosis and we are not making progesterone. If we are are in periods of long fasting while our cycle is on it throws off our progesterone levels which is why some women complain of irregular periods, hair loss and this may even cause infertility in some women. This doesn't mean you shouldn't fast at all when on your period but rather; implement Intermittent fasting vs Extended (prolonged) fasting is encouraged during this time.

*Women 40 to 55- Which happens to by my age category and she explains that as we age our estrogen & progesterone levels start to go down. The same applies to us as to where we should only do intermittent fasting while on our cycle. Those days of 21-28 of the cycle month. We need to make sure our adrenals are strong during this time and we can build these hormones by consuming certain foods during this time of the month. Some examples would be beans, rice, squash, potatoes, citrus and tropical fruit.

Fasting Spiritually - Fasting With God-

I mentioned in a previous chapter that my father was a Pastor and my experience early on with fasting was for spiritual reasons. It was to deny the flesh and to get closer to God. This was extremely hard for me as a pre-teen/ teenager and was kind of a taboo subject when my dad would mention it or if he would call a church wide fast. I honestly hated it and would cheat by eating when I went to school. I think I was just too young to understand or to make the spiritual connection. Even into my adult years, it seems like my view of fasting was to incorporate it with prayer if you really needed God to do something major in your life or to bring you through a major crisis. I think mentally I viewed it as God being my genie if I fasted when I needed something major done in my life. As a Christian I am ashamed to admit this but it's the God's honest truth.

The turn-

When I reached my 30lb mark of weight loss, I noticed that it got a bit harder to lose the last 20lbs. I had plateaued again and I just felt stuck a little. This was when I hit the 170's to 165 lb bracket. I begin to hit the gym more because I knew that would help me drop the pounds. On one particular week I decided to hit the gym more and this was my gym with the intense scientific work- outs. I increased my workouts to 5 days a week and eliminated the outside walks. My goal was to just workout hard to drop the pounds quicker! Well, I'm in my late forties and that kicked my butt! That type of workout was too strenuous on my body. I actually injured myself and had to take a full week off from working out.

During that week of rest, I was initially down and upset because that was a setback for me. This is when I decided to settle myself and give it to God. Now I was used to fasting and that was not a problem; just as I was a woman of prayer daily.

However, I never really mentally connected the two until this. One afternoon, I cried out to him about my frustration with the process. I told him that I realized that I had been trying to lose the weight in my own strength, in my own might. I acknowledged that I was stuck and needed his help. That afternoon, I carved out time just to sup with him. I yielded my mind, body and my struggle to him. I told him of how I needed help saying no to my flesh sometimes when I was tempted to indulge too much into foods, I shouldn't have during my feeding window. I cried out to him for strength and in those moments when I was tempted to overdo it - you know to eat the extra serving; I was able to crush crave the with God's help and continued focus on the goal.

Psalms 34: verses 8-10

Taste and see that the Lord is good; blessed is the one who takes refuge in him. Fear the Lord, you his holy people, for those who fear him lack nothing, the lions may grow weak and hungry, but those who seek the Lord lack no good thing.

I would also find myself praying for others that are fasting and struggling. I think overall the combination of prayer and fasting made me more sensitive to the needs of others and not to be so self-centered on my own desires.

"Fasting turns each moment of craving into a prayer of intense dependence" Gary Rohrmayer

Benefits of Fasting

What does it improve?

As mentioned, fasting has been in existence for many years and there has been countless research done on the affects that fasting has on the human body. I want to just mention a few benefits of fasting in addition to **weight loss** that have been backed by science and ways it's been beneficial to many.

Fasting:

Promotes blood sugar control by reducing insulin resistance

Promotes better health by fighting inflammation

Can enhance heart health by improving blood pressure, triglycerides as well as cholesterol levels

May boost cognitive performance (Mental Clarity) - I remember the day that I noticed a sudden increase in mental clarity. One of my many hats is that I do technical support for a publishing company and the position is really a complex one. Or should I say the job is very technical and things are constantly changing and updating and we're expected to keep up and remember it all! I had been fasting for 3 to 4 months and was getting the hang of it. I recall talking to a client on the phone and I was explaining how to resolve her technical issue, it's like something clicked in my brain! I don't mean to sound weird here but I honestly felt such a sense of confidence and just felt like my technical skills for the job had improved. In times past, I really struggled with the position and often needed to reach out for help. I noticed it the entire day with client after client - I was just able to diagnose, navigate through the systems and solve clients' issues better than I had over the past year of working there. I still work there on a part-time basis and the improved mental clarity is something I still experience.

Is known for improving A1C numbers for type II diabetics

Improvements to skin; better elasticity, tougher skin

May aid in cancer prevention and increase the effectiveness of chemotherapy

Side Effects of Fasting - Things to watch for

While it's important to share how fasting benefits us, it's also essential to share some things to watch out for and I want to encourage you not to panic and to press through the process.

Diarrhea - can occur because of over secretion of water and salts in the GI tract. Within the first 3 weeks I experienced diarrhea and honestly, I was a little concerned and wanted to quit fasting. However, I kept thinking about how much I wanted to lose the weight and just feel better so I ignored it and noticed it was not there to stay. Several things can trigger this such as drinking liquids that contain caffeine. So for us coffee drinkers or if you're drinking tea with caffeine, just be aware that you can experience diarrhea in the first few weeks.

Headaches - can also occur as you begin fasting. This is usually just because your body is adjusting. Its transitioning from the junk food; the foods high in salt - to a lower salt diet. Please don't allow a few headaches in the beginning to cause you to give up. I would take an over-the-counter pain killer to cure the headache and just keep moving. Eventually the headaches subsided.

Dizziness - is something experienced because of dehydration. Be sure you're getting in enough water. A rule of thumb with water is to drink half of your body weight in ounces. A way to add in salt so we aren't dehydrated is to add some Pink Himalayan salt to your water or you can add a little sea salt to some bone broth. Personally, I would only experience dizziness when I was doing a 48 or 72-hour fast but knew how to correct it with adding electrolytes.

Constipation - The amount of times we have bowel movements decrease when we are in our fasting windows and this is especially true when doing longer-extended fast. Increasing the fiber intake and getting in the fruit and vegetables when you're in the feeding window helps with this. Especially the leafy green vegetables. A good spinach salad is sure to help keep one regular. Another tip to counteract the constipation and to get things moving is to sip on cups of hot water throughout the day.

Muscle cramps/ spasms - I was a little alarmed when my right eye began to twitch a couple of weeks after starting OMAD. Fasting professionals explain that if we are low in magnesium, muscle cramps can be common with fasting especially those with diabetes. Some helpful tips for this is soak in Epsom salts or using magnesium oil directly to the skin should solve this issue. I did some research and found I needed to be sure I was getting in electrolytes.

Electrolytes - are necessary because when fasting we cut off the source of electrolytes that we generally get from food. To replace electrolytes when fasting - especially when doing OMAD or a prolonged fast. There are electrolyte powders you can buy to add to your water or sip on bone broth; as well as other things on the market that will not break your fast. However, I kept it simple and would sip on water I made as previously mentioned. It contained pink Himalayan salt as well as some other ingredients. This was successful with subsiding the spasms I experienced.

Heartburn - Be sure and keep moving after your meal. Its a good idea to stay active or possibly just doing something around the house after eating. Immediately lying down after the meal can cause heart burn.

Crankiness - Yes, being hungry can make us cranky. Some of us in the fasting world call it HANGRY! This does not happen every day, but its experienced more in the beginning of your fasting. Also if work may be stressful, you may find yourself getting easily agitated while fasting. The more experienced we become with fasting, we can learn to adjust to the idea of fasting in our minds. As fasting becomes normal, and we practice it daily; we learn to control the crankiness and how we respond to others while fasting.

As you join the online fasting communities you may see several acronyms while others are posting or discussing their fasting experiences and you may be wondering "what in the world" are they talking about? I wanted to share these with you so you're not confused while in these groups.

Fasting Lingo - Acronyms in the fasting world

> **IF=intermittent fasting**
> **SAD=standard American Diet**
> **OMAD=one meal a day**
> **NSV=non scale victories**
> **HIIT=high intensity interval training**
> **SW=starting weight**
> **CW-=current weight**
> **GW=goal weight**

HW=highest weight
ADF=alternate day fasting
TMAD= 2 meals a day
EF= extended fasting
ACV= apple cider vinegar

"Health and Healing Follow Fasting" Jenetzen Franklin

Participation:

In the space provided below:

Take some time to write down which method of fasting you would like to start with and why.

_____

_____

_____

_____

_____

What are 3 important takeaways from this chapter that you feel will help you most when starting out?

_____

_____

_____

7.

Fuel Up

YOU'RE STARVING! NOW What? You've just completed your first fast and maybe you can hardly think straight because you're just ready to eat! Maybe you're even a little hangry and no one can talk to you right now! You've exercised great discipline by abstaining from food and you've fasted for 12, 16, 20 or more hours; depending on your experience level and you are ready to dig in! So what do you eat?

Since we have discussed fasting in detail, I want to share with you the importance of your food choices during your feeding window; especially if your goal is to lose weight. First, I would like to ease your mind a little by saying this is a journey and things won't always be perfect. Think of it as a marathon and not a sprint. You aren't going to always cross the T's and dot the I's.

Although there is room for grace because we don't always get it right; I don't want to make light of the importance of properly refueling your body as you break your fast.

We all have heard for years that nutrition; specifically meaning what we put in our mouths; by far - out weighs everything else in the quest to lose weight. Some may disagree but what we eat is more important than how long you stay on the treadmill or how many push-ups or burpees we can do. I have personally found this to be true based upon my own personal dieting failures.

So many of us over the years have spent countless hours in the gym and can't figure out why we haven't lost any weight; or have noticed that we are just maintaining our current weight. You can workout until your face turns blue or bright red, or purple; but if you're leaving the gym and eating pancakes or pizza like I was (in the early days); you won't achieve the results you are seeking.

Breaking your fast-

During the first meal after breaking your fast, its imperative that we don't eat foods that are going to be too harsh on our digestive system. I know - all you could think about during the last few hours of your fast was gobbling down pizza or burgers. However; I want to caution you to gently move into your eating window to avoid digestive issues such as gas, bloating or heartburn from eating the wrong foods after your body has been on a reset. I want you to think about someone that is recovering from an injury. For example, a person that is recovering from a back surgery. Once they are home and are able to move about; I can guarantee you they aren't thinking about doing jumping jacks or wind sprints. They are concentrating on moving slowly and not over exerting themselves. There is a process to recovery and moving gently through the process is essential to avoid relapse or re-injury. While I know we cannot literally compare breaking a fast to a person recovering from a serious injury, I think you get my point. Take it easy and slow as you enter your feeding window.

I wanted to share some suggestions with you of how you can break your fast gently and the why behind it. As I was learning to fast, I wanted to be sure I was doing this thing properly. So I was always listening, watching and researching for answers. A few things I learned and put into practice was to enter my feeding window with **bone broth**. Bone broth is a liquid that contains brewed bones and connective tissue from animals such as cows, chickens, bison, lamb and even fish bones. There are several benefits to drinking bone broth. It can be rich in iron, vitamins A & K, fatty acids, selenium, zinc and manganese. Bone broth can be beneficial to protecting our joints, fight osteoarthritis, aid us in sleep and support weight loss. Many people make their own broth and there are countless recipes online for you to dive into the process of making it. Personally, I never had the time and found a couple of quality brands I could buy a my local grocery store. I was able to find a good brand that came in powder packets and I just had to add my hot water. This was really convenient and cost effective; especially if I didn't want to drink an entire cup. I could use half the packet and drink half a cup of broth. So even if its just a few sips before your meal, get in the habit of slowly refeeding your body.

Another suggestion is to consume foods that are high in water content. This is to help aid in hydrating the body. Most of us only think of drinking water to hydrate the body. However, there are several fruits and vegetables that are high in water content. Some examples of these are: **watermelon, honeydew melon, cantaloupe, strawberries, pineapple, peaches, oranges, bell peppers, broccoli, celery, cucumbers, lettuce and zucchini.** When selecting fruit, be sure and minimize citrus fruit so its not too acidic on the stomach. Our goal is to avoid being dehydrated.

I also often broke my fast with eggs. **I would switch things up during the week between the bone broth, fruit or some cheesy scrambled eggs.** I would consume a little just as my feeding window opened and maybe within 30 to 60 minutes after, (depending on my hunger level) I would eat the meal I had planned for that day.

Speaking of the main course - Regardless to how many times you are planning to eat within your feeding window; If at all possible, prepare your meals ahead of time and have it waiting on you; so that you don't just grab the first piece of food in sight! Knowing exactly what you're going to eat keeps you prepared, can yield better weight loss results and keeps you more confident with the process of fasting.

Deciding what to Eat - What I learned in earlier years

In one of my many quest to lose weight I learned the term "whole food". And at that time the term was new to me; just as it may be for you. I thought I was eating right while on previous diets; Especially if I was counting my calories or points as instructed by the local weight loss chain. I felt I could eat whatever I wanted as long as it was within my calorie allowance or within my allotted points for the day. I thought a bagel for breakfast and an ice cream sandwich for snack was cool as long as I didn't go over my numbers. There were a couple of things wrong with how I was eating. First, I was basically eating junk food (empty calories) and in very little time, I was hungry again. Second, I didn't realize the bagel and ice cream sandwich were refined carbohydrates that greatly spiked my insulin level and my goal should have been to eat complex carbohydrates for better results. All the while, I couldn't figure out why it was taking me six months or more to lose a measly fifteen pounds!

At a price of forty-five dollars a month plus my grocery expenses; I was paying a lot to be misguided at a local weight loss center! The problem with those food choices is that the bread and ice cream sandwich both quickly cause a spike in blood sugar and increases the insulin in the blood stream. Although, I was counting the calories - my efforts were counterproductive because I wasn't eating the proper foods for weight loss and my overall better health.

So lets talk more in detail about how I learned to eat and how you can too.

What are whole foods? Whole foods are foods that have NOT been processed or refined as little as possible. They are foods that are largely unaltered and appear as they do in nature. They are free from additives or other artificial substances.

I was learning this information while listening to trainers and coaches and even body builders online talk about whole food. It was as if a light switched on in my head!

One trainer in particular always shared his daily meal plan and conducted Q&A sessions with the viewers. While that was taking place, I was taking notes!

He discussed eating foods such as oatmeal, brown rice, quinoa, albacore tuna, red potatoes, sweet potatoes and avocado to name a few. (Sweet potatoes on a regular basis? I love them but usually only ate them for the holidays and I loaded them with brown sugar and butter!)

See - in my mind I had prejudged him because he was a body builder with muscles in unthinkable places! I just assumed he got his physique from steroids, lifting weights like a mad man and countless servings of protein powder! But here was a guy that discouraged using supplements and additional aids to lose weight! He talked about eating whole foods, exercising daily and getting plenty of rest!

Not what I expected to hear from a competitive body builder!

I learned it was time to stop buying the low-fat frozen meals that are advertised daily in the media. Instead, I learned how to read the nutritional label so I could see the loads of sodium they contained! And if we're honest with ourselves, they don't even taste great and we're still hungry after eating them. Some other whole foods I began to explore preparing were fresh green beans, broccoli, asparagus, cauliflower, Bok choy and the list continues. Growing up, I do recall my mom making fresh green beans and fresh collard greens and broccoli; but I also remember a lot of can vegetables and food being popped open to feed us. Today - as we learn better - it's time to do better. Heck there are so many choices today and recipes for making whole food taste delicious; you can even make rice from cauliflower vs having traditional white rice! I will also share some of my favorite recipes and meals I ate during my feeding window with you in the next chapter.

I quickly became aware of how consuming certain foods on a daily basis - such as cereal, bread and dairy were keeping me fat! Yes, milk, cheese, cottage cheese and my all-time favorite - the sugary fruity yogurt was stunting my weight loss success! Although it was hard to believe what I was hearing about all of the "healthy cereal brands"; I was willing to do something I hadn't done before. Once I cut back on some of the dairy products (including soy) I began to see results. A major reason why I was not successful in the earlier years, is the **inconsistency** that I discussed in a previous chapter. See most of us know what foods we should be eating but the question is - are we sick and tired enough to make some changes to see results?

When testing out what I was learning... I saw a drastic change because I had been eating a bowl of cereal daily or sometimes twice a day along with soy milk. The sugary yogurt and cottage cheese were my diet staples every single time I was on another journey to lose weight! Because if we pause to think about it; the television commercials program us to go out and buy the "latest low fat" items they're currently advertising. I felt I was eating wrong if I didn't have dairy products in my cart and besides, we've been taught they are full of protein! Yes some of the products do have a good source of protein but many yogurt brands on the shelf contain a lot of sugar! I knew I could purchase plain Greek yogurt without sugar or very little; but if I was going to eat yogurt... it had to taste good! So I quit yogurt among other dairy products.

I also began to do research on mucus and how it affects our bodies. I learned that the two main foods that cause mucus build up are dairy and wheat products. So the so called healthy cereal which was Multigrain with nuts and dried fruit in it along with my soy beverage was creating inflammation in my body. The dairy products contain casein and grain products contain gluten; which resulted in keeping my belly bloated and my body inflamed. Too much inflammation in the body stalls weight loss. I don't mean to scare you off here. Is my diet totally dairy and gluten free? No… but I've learned how to limit the amount of grains as well as dairy that I consume.

I encourage you to research the over production of mucus in the body caused by certain foods and how they can stunt your progress so you can make your own informed decisions.

Now I need to clarify here that during this period of my 7-year weight loss up and down cycle; I had not learned to fast yet and I still had more to learn about how to prepare whole food. I also learned more about dairy and chose to implement a little into my diet as a faster. For instance, I eat scrambled eggs 3 to 4 times per week and sometimes prepare them with cheese. However, I learned to switch from the more processed cheese in the wrapper that we used to slap on our eggs or make cheese toast with. I now enjoy a few cubes of feta or goat cheese with some kalamata olives as a snack. I also still occasionally enjoy a good quality brand of sharp cheddar cheese. I have mentioned the above to explain the importance of eating quality whole foods when you are in your feeding window.

A concise method to fueling up-

During another one of my weight loss ventures over the years I did learn and briefly implement the practice of "Macronutrient Dieting." Although I mentioned carbs, proteins and fat in the fasting chapter I feel its necessary to go into greater detail about Macros as many fasters do rely on and count their macros on a daily basis and have great success. So view this as an option just as I gave you different fasting methods to explore.

While I in no way claim to be an expert on macronutrient dieting… here is the basic concept of how it works.

Macronutrient dieting is the consumption of a carbohydrate, protein and a fat. And your body needs a lot of them which is why they are called MACRONUTRIENTS and not micronutrients (such as iron or zinc).

Macros also provide energy to your body. Each gram of carbohydrate contains 4 calories; protein contains 4 and fat 9.

Let's discuss why we need each nutrient:

WHY WE NEED CARBOHYDRATES

Carbohydrates in the form of starches and sugars are the macro nutrients required in the largest amounts. When eaten and broken down, carbohydrates provide the major source of energy to fuel our daily activities.

So if you're still thinking you can effectively lose weight or maintain weight loss by skipping the carbs entirely… you won't see sustainable results! It's all about the types of carbohydrates that we are consuming. The goal is to eat carbs that will not drastically increase our insulin levels when it's time to eat.

I think we all may have experienced depriving ourselves from all forms of carbs in a new quest to drop some pounds; only to find ourselves binging and devouring a pizza a week later because we just couldn't take it anymore!

So let's face the truth here - can we actually give up all carbohydrates forever to obtain the perfect body? No! The problem with me was that I was consuming too many as well as the wrong type of carbs.

Here is a small list of the complex carbohydrates I learned how to deliciously prepare and eat on a regular basis to help me achieve results. I am intentionally listing the foods that I would sometimes eat from the macronutrient component so that you have simple and clear examples. The last thing I want to do here is to write a book that my readers can't understand or follow.

Complex/ Starchy Carbohydrates: Quinoa, couscous, beans & lentils, legumes, sweet potatoes, brown rice, jasmine rice, Baz Matti rice, butternut squash, yams.

Carb Rich Fruits: grapefruit, apples, blueberries, oranges, black berries, strawberries, pears, bananas, pineapples, plums, mango. (Note, when trying to reduce weight - mango, bananas and melon fruit should be limited or eliminated; depending on the results you desire).

Ultimately when it comes to fruit; I usually stick to berries, such as strawberries, blue berries, black and raspberries because they are lower in sugar. However... I do sometimes enjoy pine-apple, grapes and navel oranges.

Low carb vegetables: (high in nutrients) Broccoli, kale, asparagus, spinach, salad greens, tomatoes, mustard/collard greens (without fatty meat) green/red peppers, onions, mushrooms, cucumbers, zucchini, green beans, peas, cauliflower and kale salad.

WHY WE NEED PROTEINS:

The proteins we consume as a part of our diet are broken down in the gut to amino acids. The body can use these amino acids in 3 main ways:

*   As building blocks in the production of new proteins needed for growth and repair of tissues, making essential hormones and enzymes and supporting immune function.
*   As an energy source.
*   As starting materials in the production of other components needed by the body.

All proteins in the body are made of up to 20 different amino acids. Eight of these are described as "essential", which means that the food we eat must contain protein capable of supplying them.

The other amino acids can be synthesized by the liver if not provided by the diet.

Protein in the diet that comes from animal sources contains all of the essential amino acids needed, whereas plant sources of protein do not. However, by eating a variety of plant sources, the essential amino acids can be supplied.

I am careful to clarify here that meat is not the one and only protein source. I have encountered many vegans & vegetarians that get an adequate supply of protein without eating meat. One can also obtain adequate amounts of protein needed daily from other food sources. In addition, as you join online fasting groups, you will find there are many fasters who are meeting their weight loss goals as they incorporate their vegan, vegetarian and even pescatarian lifestyles with fasting.

Here is a list of Proteins: Eggs, Whey protein, (protein powder supplement), chicken breast, Salmon (wild Alaskan), turkey breast, canned tuna, (solid white), nuts, (walnuts, almonds, pecans), pumpkin seeds, tofu, seitan, top round steak (grass fed if possible) flank steak (grass fed), cod fish, rainbow trout, Greek yogurt (with little or no sugar).

FAT EXPLAINED:
To conclude the nutrient of fat… it's very important to know that there are 3 different types of fat.

Saturated fats: are found in foods like meat, butter, and cream (animal sources).

Unsaturated fats: found in foods like olive oil, avocados, nuts and canola oil (plant sources).

Trans fats: found in commercially produced baked goods, snack foods, fast foods and some margarine. Just a note about trans-fats, you need not consider those prepackage foods your friends if weight loss is your goal.

Despite what we've been taught over the years, fat can be good for us. The goal with fat is to consume fat that will keep us sustained longer when we enter the fasting window again. Some examples of this would be:

Avocados
Cheese (may have to limit your portions)
Dark Chocolate
Whole Eggs
Fatty Fish
Nuts
Chia Seeds
Olive Oil
Butter (grass fed is suggested)
MCT Oil
Avocado Oil

And when it comes to using oils, although it may be difficult to retrain old habits; try to **avoid using these plant/vegetable base oils** as they can be high in omega 6 which can lead to chronic inflammation in the body. To list these would be **soybean oil, corn oil, cotton seed oil, canola, sesame, grape seed, peanut and rice bean oil**.

Since we've learned why we need carbs, proteins, fats and explored how they work… there is actually a more detailed process of coordinating these 3 macronutrients into your daily routine of food intake. This is termed as **"Counting Macros"**. While I chose not to count macros or calories during my feeding window, I think it's important to at least briefly explain how counting macros works and you can make the decision as to if you want to include this in your regimen or not. Many health professionals and fitness gurus will say one cannot be successful at weight loss without calculating their macros; but honestly for me… at this point I was sick of counting and calculating. However, people who thrive on structure may find that counting macros is ideal for their health goals. So, counting or not counting boils down to a personal choice and many fasters are successful with both methods.

Here's an example by Dr. & Dietitian Jillian Kubala of how to calculate macronutrients for a 2,000-calorie diet consisting of 40% carbs, 30% protein and 30% fat.

However, first know that: when starting out and endeavoring to counting macros, it's easy to feel overwhelmed but as you consistently do it, it feels natural. The most important steps in calculating macros are setting a calorie goal and macronutrient range for carbs, protein and fat that works best for you.

Then, log your food intake and aim to stay within your macros by eating a diet rich in fresh produce, healthy fats, complex carbs and protein sources.

So here it goes - Here's the example:

Carbs:
- 4 calories per gram
- 40% of 2,000 calories = 800 calories of carbs per day
- Total grams of carbs allowed per day = 800/4 = 200 grams

Proteins:
- 4 calories per gram
- 30% of 2,000 calories = 600 calories of protein per day
- Total grams of protein allowed per day = 600/4 = 150 grams

Fats:
- 9 calories per gram
- 30% of 2,000 calories = 600 calories of protein per day
- Total grams of fat allowed per day = 600/9 = 67 grams

In this scenario, your ideal daily intake would be 200 grams of carbs, 150 grams of protein and 67 grams of fat.

Why counting can be beneficial:

To count macros, determine your calorie and macronutrient needs, then log macros into an app or food journal.

Counting macros may ensure that your macronutrient needs are being met.

Counting macros can increase your awareness of the quality and amount of food you are consuming.

So that's macronutrient dieting in a quick synopsis should you choose to incorporate this strategy in your feeding window. There are many websites and bloggers that discuss macros in detail. And trust me as you enter the fasting world online you will get varying opinions as to if counting macros is absolutely necessary or not. Just as you will hear that many only lose weight by counting and that some simply fast and lose the weight without so much structure.

Processed Foods - Should We Eat Them?

So, we know what whole foods are and some examples have been given. I am sure by now you're probably already confirming mentally what you like and don't like when it comes to whole food. So, let's dive into **processed food -** processed foods as explained by Sport and Exercise Scientists Jack Wilson - are foods that are processed in order to improve taste (this is the process of optimizing food to be discussed in a later chapter), increase shelf life and to make them look appealing. Food is also processed to make them more consistent in shape; as well as making them easier to package and transport to stores. Another important fact about the processing of food is they are processed to increase or decrease certain nutritional values. This is good news for food manufactures but not for you and me.

See the problem with processed foods is that many of them are altered by manufactures and can be addictive to us as consumers. Think about the time you ate the doughnut or a huge glazed honey bun you picked up at the convenience store when you went to buy gasoline. You gobbled it down while driving and by the time you arrived to your destination, your taste buds were screaming for more; or better yet you were probably craving salty potato chips. Many processed foods lack nutrients but invade our bodies with artificial preservatives, flavorings and coloring and have been linked by researchers with adverse side effects ranging from headaches to cancer. I can remember when my boys were small and were screaming for me to buy the fruity cereal with the rainbow of colors. I wasn't health conscious at all back then but I just knew there was something about that cereal that wasn't right. Mind you - it even had an inky taste in my opinion.

There is so much more that can be discussed regarding processed food but I simply want to raise your awareness a little and to encourage you to move away from popping open a can of vegetables because its quick and convenient and look more into fresh or frozen vegetables and whole foods when you are making your choices.

"A Healthy Outside Starts From The Inside" Robert Urich

Participation time:

In the space provided below:

Begin to make a list of whole foods you enjoy and will be incorporating into your meals during your feeding window. Also make a list of the whole foods you have been afraid to try. With the list of foods you have been apprehensive about trying, your assignment is to check YouTube, Pinterest or just online in general for recipes that catch your attention so you can give the new food choices a chance.

<u>Whole Foods I Enjoy</u>-

_____

_____

_____

_____

_____

_____

<u>Whole Foods I'm Willing to Explore</u>-

_____

_____

_____

_____

_____

_____

8.

Refuse to eat boring food!

JUICY MEATBALLS, FINGER Lickin' Chicken Wings, pan seared Salmon and Shrimp - kept my taste buds roaring! Now that we've discussed fasting and refueling our bodies in great detail; I want to share some meals or meal ideas of foods that I ate. Meals I actually prepared while on the journey. The last thing I want to do is to be fake or phony about what I ate. Besides, after abstaining from food for 18 hours plus, I wanted to eat scrumptious tasty meals but also something that would sustain me.

I previously mentioned a list of saturated(good) fats and I definitely added some to my food selections as I planned my meals. So just be forewarned I'm not going to give you a bunch of salad ideas although I did incorporate salad into some of my meals. I also want you to know that I'm a busy entrepreneur and did not always have time to prepare a full scale home cooked meal. First, I will share some of my favorite meals that I ate during my first 30lbs of weight loss. After the first 30lbs, just as having to kick up the exercise, I had to change up my food selections a little to see more results which catapulted me to the 50lb goal. So I will break the favorite meals into two categories and explain how I prepared them.

Although when fasting and refueling you can pretty much eat what you want when it's time to eat; when beginning I knew from past experiences, I needed to cut some things out.

So, If I was in the mood for breakfast as my first meal at noon or 1pm. Here's I would eat:

Breakfast Ideas -

Simple Breakfast:
    scrambled eggs with sharp cheddar cheese
    two slices of bacon
fresh pineapple slices

Another option was to switch up the meat and the fruit if I was bored with bacon.

    Scrambled eggs with sharp cheddar cheese
    2 sausage patties or the old fashion Uncle Jones Pride Sausage
grapes - usually a hand-full

Hearty Breakfast:
If I was in the mood for something a little more heavy on the stomach, here's what I would make:

    Sweet potatoes (without the sugar)
    scrambles eggs minus the cheese
    sautéed spinach & onions

Here is how I prepared the sweet potatoes. I had two variations of this depending on what I was in the mood for. If I wanted a little crunch, I would cube the fresh sweet potatoes in chunks.

After cubing them I would spray or coat my baking sheet with olive oil. Then lightly rub a little coconut oil on the potatoes and a pinch of salt and bake until I got them to the tenderness I desired. When coming out of the oven, I would sprinkle them with cinnamon.

Another variation of my breakfast sweet potatoes would be to first to wash and poke the fresh sweet potato. I would then coat it with coconut oil and place the potato on a large piece of aluminum foil and bake for 80 to 90 minutes with the oven temperature at 400 degrees. I baked them this long because I wanted the potato to be soft and full of rich flavor. After baking, I would cut the sweet potato in half and top it with a little butter and cinnamon.

Notice here regarding the sweet potatoes; that I did not add sugar to either variation. I had learned to appreciate the natural sweet taste of the potato without adding refined sugar or other sweeteners.

Sautéed Spinach

I would generally keep my cast iron skillet on the stove and I would coat it with olive or coconut oil and heat it. I would then add thinly sliced onions and caramelize them. After the onions were nice and brown, I added a little Pink Himalayan salt and freshly washed spinach. I would sauté to my liking so the spinach wasn't too soggy and plate it with the eggs.

Large Egg Omelet

I was usually starving when it was time to eat so if I was craving an omelet, I would heat the pan with butter and coat it really well so the eggs did not stick to the pan. I would use 3 to 4 eggs depending on my hunger level. This was a hearty meal for me and I would usually add sausage crumbles, onion, bell pepper, cherry tomatoes and cheese.

I was definitely full and it kept me going until my second meal of the day.

Shrimp & Eggs

When I was feeling a little fancy, I would sauté shrimp and onions together in a pan with a little coconut oil. I would usually use a little old bay seasoning to give the shrimp a little kick and some garlic. I would plate the shrimp with 3 scrambled eggs and it was delicious!

Eggs & Zesty Salmon

When I was feeling a little bougie, I would pan sear a chunk of wild caught salmon. I used a little Pink Himalayan salt and lemon pepper seasoning to give it the zestiness I was looking for. I occasionally would add a little fresh rosemary. Plated with my scrambled eggs this dish did not disappoint! I was feeling a little high and mighty when I ate this combination as my first meal of the day.

The breakfast choices listed above were filling foods to me and kept me until my next meal. I usually ate my breakfast of choice no later that 1pm and my last meal of the day was usually between 4:30 and 6pm depending on my hunger level and my evening time activity.

Lunch or Dinner Ideas-

Friends, I want to reassure you that you can eat well when your feeding window opens. So below are some meals I prepared as a lunch or dinner meal depending on my refeeding time.

Lemon Dill Salmon Burgers - Grilled Shrimp Skewers & Veggies

OK, this meal is not as complicated as it seems so don't be intimated by the title. While there are plenty of recipes for salmon burgers online. I did not hand make these burgers. I would go to my local grocery store and purchase the burgers from the seafood deli. They were large thick burgers and cost about $5 each. I usually purchased 4 at a time so I could pull them from the freezer and eat as my taste buds longed for one. This was simple to prepare by lightly browning in a skillet until warm through out. When done, I would drizzle a creamy garlic sauce that I bought in the same seafood department of my grocery store. As for the shrimp, I would peel and remove the tails and put them on long skewers along with chunks of zucchini, I would grill just long enough to darken the shrimp but was careful not to over cook the zucchini chunks.

This was really a favorite meal me and I honestly felt like royalty when I sat down to eat it. I was just so good and different from the greasy carb rich foods I had been eating before. If you are a seafood lover, its a great meal to add to your selections.

Feta Burger& Sweet Kale Salad

As you can probably tell, I use my grill a lot. Several times a week to be honest. So the burgers of course are grilled. This is a quick simple meal for sure. I season the burger with something a little robust from my pantry and grill the burger to my liking so its still juicy inside. There are no hard dry burgers in my house! Once the burger is done I plate it with feta cheese chunks and bold strong olives that I pickup from the olive bar at my local grocer. The sweet kale salad is also purchased from the grocery store. The greens are a mixture of dark greens and cabbage slaw and can be found in the fresh vegetable area of the store. The brands usually available are Eat Smart and Taylor Farms. The dressing is a sweet poppy seed dressing and it comes with a package of cranberries and roasted pumpkin seeds. Its such a great combination especially if you often crave salty and sweet together.

Sesame Ginger & Teriyaki Wings

For these chicken wings, I usually buy whole wings and cut the tips off and separate the flat from the drum. When I can get wings already bagged and separated, of course I take advantage of that. Once again, I grill the wings or if hubby is home, I have him put them in the smoker! Oh! - smoked chicken wings are the best when I can have that luxury. Either way, smoked or grilled I take an easy route and drizzle them with a sauce I picked up at my grocery store. This sauce is gluten free and is made by BIBIBOP Asian Grill. The flavor is sesame ginger teriyaki and the flavor is AMAZING! It can actually be used for stir frying, as marinade or as a dipping sauce. I plated these wings with some broccoli and I felt like I was in Asian heaven!

Sweet n Sour Meatballs & Veggies

For some reason, I desired meatballs a lot for dinner after fasting. Depending on my time, I would make home-made meat balls based upon on the meat I had in my freezer. It would vary from ground turkey to ground chuck if I had any. I would season the meat to my liking; brown them a little on top of the stove and finish baking in the oven to be sure they were cooked thoroughly. If I absolutely had no time to make home made meatballs, I would pickup a pack of frozen ones and get the same results. I would plate them and cover with sweet and sour dipping sauce from my local grocery store. The brand of sauce I used was Kikkoman. I'm a huge fan of broccoli so I would often enjoy the meatballs with sautéed broccoli and caramelized onions. Of course, you could use spinach or which ever vegetable is your go to veggie.

Spicy Sautéed Shrimp & Asparagus

As mentioned at the beginning of this chapter, I said I would honestly tell you what I ate during the journey and I'm doing just that. I enjoyed these meals during my feeding window while doing the 16:8 or OMAD fasting methods. I occasionally added a garlic knot to my meal(if I was in the mood for bread) and still lost weight.

I didn't eat not one cardboard tasting rice cake or sit and count hundreds of calories a day to do it!

So on to this shrimp and asparagus. I would oven roast the asparagus by using a few tablespoons full of olive oil, season with a little salt and garlic. Yes I love garlic! I would roast them with the oven temperature at 425 degrees and bake for 12 minutes. As for the shrimp, I would peel and season with Old Bay seasoning and sautée in a pan with onions and sometimes mushrooms. Talk about delish!

Seafood Rice Bowl

When I was wanting something hearty or just in the mood for heavier carbs, I would prepare forbidden black rice and season it to my liking. I would often use chicken or beef broth when I boiled the rice. The seafood I would add was shrimp, scallops and salmon chunks. I would lightly season the seafood to taste. Of course I added some short broccoli florets that I pan seared separately. This was a nice colorful dish and was sure to keep me full. Once the bowl was prepared, I would drizzle with my creamy garlic seafood sauce. Although I did not count calories, since I was eating rice, I knew it was higher in calorie content than most dishes I ate so I would do OMAD on days that I prepared this meal. I knew I would see a little weight gain if I ate a breakfast meal and this hearty rice bowl all in the same day. Of course my husband loved this one because it was rich in flavor and heavy on his tummy!

Grilled Chicken & Roasted Veggies

Some days, I just kept dinner simple. I would season chicken breast to my liking and grill the breast until they were rich and smoky. Something I forgot to mention is that regardless to which meat I'm grilling I would baste the meat with Italian salad dressing so the meat was always moist and never dry and over cooked on the grill. One thing I detest about grilling meat is burnt BBQ!

When I used the grill especially since it was a gas grill, I nursed whatever I was cooking. I would also cut up broccoli, brussels sprouts, onions and cauliflower and season to my liking. One of my favorite seasonings to coat on these veggies was smoked paprika!

The smoked paprika that I was able to get from a store in my area which was Bulk Nation was the best. The flavor of this fresh paprika was just superior to the store brands of smoked paprika.

Zucchini & squash noodles

As a child and even into my adult years, I did not care for these vegetables. They always seemed to be tasteless and mushy! It actually wasn't until I started fasting that I learned to prepare zucchini and squash properly and still have them taste good. See what is good to know is that both zucchini and summer squash are considered water content vegetables. They both contain over 90 % water which means you can't cook it too long. I invested in a vegetable cutter and it made nice spiral spaghetti like noodles with these vegetables. I would season with olive oil, salt, lemon pepper and lightly saute in a pan for just 3 minutes or so. I wanted them to keep some of their crunchiness. This was so good, one week, I ate these veggies for a week straight! I would just change up my meat choice.

Hopefully from sharing the foods I enjoyed above that I have assured that you can eat good while eating whole food. You no longer have to be a slave to rice cakes and low fat prepackaged foods. Although I selected frozen meatballs on occasion for the convenience, I tried to keep my process food conception to a minimum.

I made the decision to switch from refined carbohydrates as my breakfast and dinner choices to foods that were whole and more sustaining. For instance, in previous years I would eat sugary oatmeal, pancakes or cereal for breakfast as my first meal of the day.

After learning of how to fast, the goal was to avoid consuming simple carbohydrates because they would quickly spike my insulin levels. Simple carbohydrates also left me feeling bloated, heavy and foggy. I had more energy from whole foods.

However because we aren't perfect people and sometimes we are going to desire bread, I would enjoy a roll or slice of pumpernickel bread with my meal. I was cautious though and limited my bread intake to once or twice a week. I simply just could not eat bread anymore on a daily basis if I was going to really lose the weight! As you begin to reset your taste buds, you actually won't desire the bread among other things as often as before.

As a side note: regarding any **sauces** listed above that came from a jar in my local grocery store, I would choose a sauce that had **5 grams or less of sugar**. This was a trial and error experience and I learned rather quickly which ones I liked and did not. I can truly say I had fun and enjoyed experimenting with my meals. I am a big fan of our large gas grill and would use it several times per week. If you are not into grilling or don't own one; you can also invest in an Instapot or a Ninja Foodi to assist you with quick but delicious meals. There are so many new cooking gadgets available to us today that can make cooking faster which also takes away the excuse to be in the drive thru lines. Friends, please don't be afraid to season your food! I was a big fan of using herbs and spices especially to season my meat prior to grilling. Some of the spices I used to season my food with were: **fresh garlic, sea salt, onion powder, garlic powder, garlic salt, smoked paprika, fresh rosemary (great for pork), thyme and I also bought combination seasonings from my grocery store such as lemon pepper, jerk seasoning** and more.

It also helps when your family is on board. I am thankful that my husband was easy going and would eat whatever I prepared. In the beginning though; I had to make him some starchy mashed potatoes, yellow rice; or he needed bread on a regular basis. However, as he saw me making progress with my weight loss - he greatly reduced the starchy foods and would eat everything I prepared for dinner.

The Change Up-

As I continued in my journey my progress stalled after I got to the 30 pound mark or so. The weight loss community would call this a plateau. It was frustrating for several weeks because the scale didn't move up or down. I learned to change things up with my food choices and will explain this in more detail.

Because my ultimate goal was to lose 50lbs, I couldn't just stop at 30lbs. Although I was slimmer and felt better, I knew there was more for me to accomplish. Especially because I could still see belly and back fat that I was still unhappy with. So when I hit the 170's range; down from 207 and things seem to stall, I had to evaluate where I could cut back and how I could increase the workouts.

In the fasting chapter I briefly discussed **Alternate Day Fasting (ADF)** So when deciding to change things up within my feeding window, I made two changes that took me to my goal. With implementing ADF, I would eat 1 to 2 meals on my feeding day and after the 2 meals I would go into fasting mode for an entire day and refuel the morning of the third day.

On the morning of my feeding window, I was famished and ready eat however, I kept my food selections simple because I had become more focused on meeting my goals. I felt great in my body and had become a more experienced faster so I felt like I had really taken on the mindset that I was eating to live and nor longer living to eat. So I will share with you below some of my ADF food selections on the feeding days as I took my progress to the next level.

First, here is an example of what my schedule was like: I would eat breakfast on Monday at 10:30 am and have my last meal at 4:30 that afternoon. I would then enter fasting mode by fasting all day on Tuesday and refueling again on Wednesday of that week.

Also, on the feeding days, I started to curtail my sugar intake. I just knew there were some areas I could cut back some to really get me to my goal.

For instance, I cut out the sweet fruit I was consuming. I decided to stop religiously buying the pineapples and grapes every week. I had to switch it up and then started purchasing fruit that did not have the high sugar content.

I substituted them for **black berries, blue berries and straw-berries**. Switching to fresh berries was a better choice because they were lower in sugar and quick to pickup and eat. Again, just like the sweet potato I mentioned earlier, I learned to enjoy the natural sweetness of the fruit. I have to be honest here and say giving up the pineapple and grapes was a little hard for me but my taste buds adjusted in a week or two.

ADF Food Selections-

Breakfast Ideas:

Cheese eggs or a large omelet along with berries of my choice.

Lunch & Dinner Ideas:

As far as my meat selections I started to cut back on how often I ate chicken wings, bacon and the frozen meatballs. I would limit them to once a week or every two weeks. I began to incorporate more fish into my meals. The fish would be pan seared or baked vs fried. My fish selections were **salmon, flounder, cod and Mahi Mahi.** I would also incorporate **shrimp** and **scallops** into my meals.

My vegetable choices didn't change much. I would still prepare tasty **broccoli, brussels sprouts, cauliflower, asparagus, spinach and hearty salads**. However, I limited how often I ate sweet pota-toes and rice. As mentioned, we do need carbohydrates to fuel the body. I was just more focused on my goal and had to cut back where necessary.

I know at this point it sounds as if I had gone Keto, but I had not. I did however research Keto recipes and tweaked them to my liking.

Honestly, I don't think I could ever fully convert to "Ketoism" because I personally did not find it to be sustainable. I know many differ from my opinion but its just that - for me Keto was not sustainable.

Remember, what we do to lose the weight it what we have to keep doing for it to be sustainable. So I would only adapt to a keto diet (short term) when I knew I was over doing it on the sugary fruit.

As mentioned throughout this book, you will find that you have to find a balance that works for you regardless to if its concerning your food choices or your exercise routine.

So here are some of the meals I put together and they were mouth watering, and satisfying! I took the "don't reinvent the wheel" approach and searched for recipes online and watched many YouTube videos on low carb meals. I did however sometimes change up some of the ingredients when necessary. For instance, if I chose a recipe that contained all purpose flour or corn starch; I would switch them out for **almond or coconut flour** to give me the thickening I needed in the dish.

Seafood & Sprouts

This was a tasty combination! I would saute scallops, shrimp and onions together in a pan with my favorite seasonings. In a separate pan I would season brussel sprouts, broccoli and mushrooms. I then drizzled the veggies with avocado oil to give them a little more life before baking. These come out great and with a bit of a crunch if baking on 400 degrees for just 15 minutes or so.

****Try not to over cook your veggies so they aren't soggy and lifeless. Just combine the seafood with the veggies and its a meal to be talked about!

Chicken Cheese Wraps

So I never knew cheese wraps existed but in my search for wrap recipes, I found that I could make wraps from lettuce or cheese vs the standard tortilla wraps. While feta and goat cheese are usually my go to for cheese when I have it; these cheese wraps were the bomb! They come in cheddar or pramesean flavor and the brand is **FOLIOS**; however, I am sure there are other brands in your local grocer. The wraps are best at room temperature vs being cold directly from the fridge; and they are more pliable. **These wraps are sure to excite your mouth when adding a grilled chicken strip, a few pieces of shrimp, fresh spinach and thinly sliced cherry tomatoes. Another suggestion is to add a little sour cream or guacamole or a slice of avocado.** I just want to forewarn you, these wraps are very thin and overloading them may cause the wrap to break when trying to close it. I usually used a skewer to keep it closed as I ate the wrap. This one is will not disappoint!

Smoked Beef Brisket & Zucchini Noodles

I spiral cut the **fresh zucchini** so that it had a noodle texture like spaghetti. I then sautéed it with onion, garlic and olive oil. I used salt and pepper to taste and it was delicious! If you are not into zucchini or summer squash, you could switch this out for cauliflower. Cauliflower is actually a new craze today since many are making rice, pizza crust and much more from it.

Now on to the **corn beef brisket** - I would purchase a large beef brisket from our local butcher and we can usually get a few meals from it. The brisket comes with a tiny seasoning packet of spices. The little packet gives the brisket such a distinctive flavor, its unforgettable! Just follow the package directions for boiling the brisket. Once its done boiling, we refrigerate for at least an hour for it to cool down and then my husband smokes it and thinly slices it. Even if you don't have the ability to smoke it, it can be thinly sliced and drizzled with your favorite sauce and baked at 400 degrees for just a few minutes until the sauce is crisped on top.

Curry Chicken Soup

While, we all may have our own variations of how we make curry chicken especially for my readers from the Caribbean. They are superior for sure when it comes to curry chicken. There are many versions that can be found online so I will not go into the details of how prepare mine. I would take the completed curry chicken which is usually made with a creamy coconut sauce (or some call it gravy) and add my favorite veggies to the chicken and gravy sauce. The veggies used were broccoli, zucchini and carrots. I would avoid adding rice or potatoes to cut down on my carb intake. However, I didn't feel deprived in any way because the tender chicken chunks and hearty vegetables were definitely filling.

Because this dish is a hearty one and the coconut milk used is really rich - this would also be treated as an **OMAD** for me.

So What's for Dessert?

Although we are putting the work in and meeting goals, we're still human and I don't think any of us will forever say No to dessert on occasion. So I knew at this phase of trying to get to that final goal I had evaluate my dessert selections when I did have dessert. Since I felt like my baking skills were top notch, I could not always indulge in the desserts that I made for family the family.

So here are some choices I made for dessert:

First, a little side note- Another reason why I could not convert to "Ketoism" is because I baked a keto chocolate cake one morning and it was an unforgettable experience! I purchased the 2 types of flour, the sugar substitute recommended, and all the other pricey ingredients. I also made home made icing and the cake batter yielded about 12 jumbo chocolate cupcakes. The cupcakes were very moist and melted in my mouth; however – the flavor was horrible! I just couldn't handle the taste of the sugar substitute.

Seriously, the taste was a total turn off for me and I felt like I had been duped by the Keto world!

So I have to be honest with you when I still wanted something sweet, at least once a week or so; I had 2 go to items that satisfied me and were not as heavy and dense as a slice of cake or pie.

My dessert choices when taking things to the next level were:

Lindt Intense Orange Dark Chocolate Bar - This chocolate was smooth and just melted in my mouth! I loved the contrast of the orange flavor mixed with the dark chocolate. Here's the trick though, I would not stock it in the house. I would only go to my local grocer and pick it up when I wanted chocolate and the bar would give me about 3 to 4 servings. I never ate the entire bar in one day.

The other dessert choice was: Triple Berry Fruit Salad with Poppy Seed Dressing-

This fruit salad was really easy to make and satisfied my desire for something sweet. I simply washed and dried black berries, blue berries and diced strawberries. I also picked up a jar of poppy seeds. I then used a little honey, lime zest and lime juice. Just simply mix all the ingredients together and chill it in the fridge. A quick search online for this recipe to get the exact ratios of the ingredients; is suggested so you have the proper balance of sweet and tart. I so enjoyed the combination!

I promise you, it will satisfy that need for something sweet without the high calorie count of cake, cookies or pies.

Remember, we really no longer have the excuse of saying its too hard to eat healthy. We have countless choices that are quick and easy to prepare that will keep our taste buds excited! We don't have to settle for bland boring food just because of our goals. We just have to be willing to take the time to prepare whole foods that are good for us just as we did when we ate unhealthy. Remember, we planned the fried chicken dinners and the high carb potlucks with friends.

Trust me; you really can enjoy this journey of fasting and re - fueling the body with food that is vibrant in color, bold in taste and nourishing as you lose the weight you so desire.

"To eat is a necessity, but to eat intelligently is an art"
Francois de la Rochefoucauld

Participation time:

Hopefully from reading some of the meal examples you have an idea of the foods you will add to your palette in your feeding window.

From the list you created in the previous chapter, plan your own menus for at least seven days so that you know exactly what you're going to eat during your feeding window.

Think about what you would enjoy as a breakfast, lunch or dinner meal. Plan according to the number of meals or snacks you will include in your feeding window. Here's a chart below to help you get started.

My 7 Day Meal Plan

Meal 1: Time Meal 2: Time	Meal 1: Time Meal 2: Time
Meal 1: Time Meal 2: Time	Meal 1: Time Meal 2: Time

Meal 1: Time Meal 2: Time	Meal 1: Time Meal 2: Time
Meal 1: Time Meal 2: Time	

9.

Get your booty moving!

THE POUNDING SOUND of my heavy feet hitting the pavement; and the exhaustive panting I did while running as a beginner was something I was avoiding!

My body felt as if it was a heavy loaded dump tuck trying to move quickly down the street. I could also vividly remember fighting the thoughts in my head of giving up after the first couple minutes into a 30-minute run.

Although I had found a few fasting methods that worked for me; I knew I had to start moving outside or in the gym.

I had been fasting for about 2 months; lost 7lbs and could really see my face slimming and the bloating in my belly was decreasing some.

However, I knew if I wanted to see real results, I had to over-ride the complacency in the area of exercise. See, I knew my body. Regardless to which weight loss gimmick I had succumb to over the years; I was never successful at any of them if I did not exercise.

So although I was recalling the awful feelings of beginning again, I decided to start small. At this point in my life I was closer to 50 than I was 40. I was recovering from a back injury due to a car accident a couple of years prior and I had not exercised at all in 9 months. So I decided to just walk. I dismissed the dreaded thoughts of running and began to walk 3 to 4 evenings per week. I consistently walked and as I got more energy and strength, I increased my walking to 5 days per week. I started out walking 4 miles each time I went and eventually increased to 6 miles.

As the weeks passed I saw the pounds just fall off! I had found my formula! I was enjoying this new journey of fasting and enjoying my meals immensely during my feeding window. Fasting with the increased days per week and adding mileage was working!

Finding your groove

As I continued to walk and fast daily, I got a little bored after about 3&1/2 months of walking. I finally had more energy and I was ready to do something else! After doing a little research, I started doing HITT Workouts. I downloaded an app and ventured into something different.

HITT is defined as high intensity interval training or sprint interval training and is basically a cardiovascular exercise strategy. It consist of alternating short periods of intense anaerobic exercise with less intensive recovery periods.

So for me the HITT Workout was to walk for 3 minutes and run for 1 minute and to do several sets of this. When doing high intensity workouts, you should keep the routine within 30 minutes or less because you are literally tearing down your body.

As I incorporated the HITT routine into my weekly workouts, I decreased the amount of days I walked. So at this point I was walking 3 days and doing HITT 2 days per week.

After these workouts, I felt like I could literally feel the fat burning and melting away!

The workout felt like torture as I pushed my body to its max but later in the week when I got on the scale, it was all worth it and I was encouraged to keep going.

Another way of finding my groove was that I fell in love again with a childhood hobby that I enjoyed so much. Rollerskating!

Yes... I began roller skating again. It had been at least 10 to 15 years since I had even tried on a pair. I had to use wisdom here and be sure I was padded up and wore a helmet while skating. I was too old and had too many important things to accomplish then to be dealing with broken bones.

So I began skating on Sunday mornings while my husband rode his bike. Skating is definitely a total body workout. Skating improves heart health, strengthens our muscles and helps us burn calories. Gliding on those wheels works muscles in the legs, glutes and core. We can burn about 600 calories per hour from roller skating.

My point here is for you to grant yourself permission to have fun! To enjoy yourself as you exercise to get the pounds off. As of recent, manufactures are making skates in bright colors with flashy laces and it just makes for a more enjoyable experience. I made a weekly schedule of which days I would walk, do HITT, and skate.

Maybe your groove is zumba, long distance running or cross-fit... regardless to what it is - I encourage you not to be afraid to venture out and try new things.

Don't go it alone - joining a fitness community

If you are one that needs support to workout, then join a gym that offers group fitness classes. There are also personal trainers that may offer small group sessions if you don't care to be a part of larger group classes.

Although throughout the years I'd experienced losing and gaining weight; there was a seed of exercise that was planted in my life. I encountered some people in the earlier days that inspired and motivated me to grow. This brings me to the most memorable experience of incorporating exercise into my life at the local YMCA.

One particular morning, I met a gorgeous couple that were older than me and they both were just buff! I mean muscles popping out every-where! They stood out to me because there were very few African-American people in my area at the time. I'm sure I was noticeable to them as well because I was overweight and looked as if the equipment in the gym intimated me. We engaged in a little small talk one morning as I was leaving the gym and they encouraged me to start working out at least five days a week. During our conversation I mentioned that my endeavor was just to hop on the treadmill three days a week at 6:00am because that's all I knew to do.

In a few short weeks after meeting this couple, I noticed posters on the wall introducing new boot camp classes and running groups being held at the Y.

After getting up the nerve to join these groups, I quickly established a rapport with the trainer and members of the group. The trainer was a little short and highly energetic woman by the name of Aimee. Meeting her was like a breath of fresh air. She was funny and made exercise fun. In boot camp; I was surrounded by a group of rambunctious competitive men and women who were willing to exercise in the dark (and run through mud) at 5:00 am because it was good for our bodies and we were looking for results! The more I showed up; I was starting to see my butt lift and to see muscles form on my arms from the push-ups. Let's clarify… they were girly push-ups! And I still do girly push-ups today!

While I enjoyed her boot camps, I really found a sense of community when I joined her running group. Although in the beginning, I was slow and always finished last or second to last the group always encouraged me to keep going. I was taught techniques for running such as how to breathe and to lengthen my stride. It was important to breathe properly and pace myself so I wouldn't give up within the first few minutes. The running group had nothing but encouragement for me every step of the way!

I remember in the beginning - running and having to hold my back because it hurt so bad but I wouldn't give up. The extra weight I was carrying made running difficult. However, the more consistent I was with showing up three days a week, the faster I became and I gained more confidence. At the end of the eight-week session; I was able to run for thirty minutes without stopping! After finding my pace and settling in the run; it was like I mentally entered another world. I didn't think about my problems while running. I actually got creative ideas about my business or special projects I was working on while running. Running was like a place of escape for me; and joining that group was one of the best things I have ever done and I'm still a runner today because of it.

I have mentioned the above experiences not to boast or for you to think that the exercise was easy for me. I remember fighting back tears several times while running because my body hurt so bad. I was moving joints that had been so stagnant for a while. I even fell one day after my run and dislocated my shoulder. But I wouldn't give up! A couple of weeks after, I jogged a slower pace behind the group with my arm in a sling. I didn't decide to quit exercise all together because I got injured or because it was too hard. I saw my body transforming and I even had more energy for sex! I was loving this new me!

The Decision

Hopefully, you've mentally made the decision that you will get moving. Now its time to take some physical steps in to that direction. I encourage you to start walking for at least 30 minutes 4 to 5 days a week. If you can handle a 1-hour walk vs the 30 minutes then go for it!

However, when walking… put some real effort into it. If you are walking down the sidewalk and can scroll through your social media pages at the same time, you will see mediocre results. Your arms should be moving as well your legs and you should be walking fast enough so that its difficult to have a conversation. What I'm getting at here is… your walk shouldn't be casual. Extend those hips, swing your arms and twist that booty! A casual slow walk will yield minimal results which may cause you to quit.

If you cant get your booty moving as swiftly as you'd like to; and if you are considered morbidly obese, then obviously you may have to start at a slower pace but your consistency will pay off. You can do it! I'm cheering for you!

You have to decide today - how you will incorporate exercise into your daily schedule. Its really time to eliminate any excuses you may have if you truly want to execute some fat! We all are given the same 24 hours in the day and you just have to decide which time of day works best for you.

If joining group fitness is the route you want to take, you will notice the same faces showing up for your class and it will start to feel as if they are your supporters or accountability partners. So let your hair down! Be yourself and enjoy this new community that you have joined.

The importance of Strength Training

After I had been consistent for several months with fasting and exercise... I knew I needed to take my journey to the next level. Actually, I was a little over half way to my goal. I had reached 28lbs of fat loss but I knew I had to kick things up a notch or two. I initially tried following body weight exercises at home by streaming YouTube and I was OK with that for a few workouts. But the truth is... I don't work as hard when I'm alone when it comes to the weights, push-up, burpees and all of the stuff that comes along with that. Here was another area where I needed a sense of accountability, a sense of community; you know someplace - to show up to so I would actually complete the routines. Completing a strength training workout alone for me was challenging. I would get through maybe half of the reps and decided it hurt too bad and told myself I would start again tomorrow. See I had been accustom to accountability through group exercise in my earlier years and that was the best fit for me to see results.

You may be a self-starter and even a finisher when it comes to exercise and if you can do the push-ups, lift the dumbbells and squat it out alone... that is awesome! Keep it up !

Personally, I needed help so I joined a gym in my area that actually offered scientific based workouts. Joining Orange Theory - was definitely something new for me and even more challenging than the boot camps from my earlier years. It was a one-hour full body workout focused on endurance, strength and power. The workouts are considered heart rate based interval training, which burns more calories than traditional exercise. The intensity is based on your own individual heart rate zones, making the workout effective for any and all fitness levels. Talk about taking it to the max; when I left those classes, I was exhausted and couldn't speak. I would often just sit in my car to recover a bit before driving home! Honestly, I hated hitting the button on the app to reserve a class and dreaded it all the way to class but felt great as soon as I hit the water rowing machine. The more I attended classes there and got to know all of the trainers, I was hooked! I had discovered another effective way to get my booty moving!

I want to encourage you to not just settle for cardio workouts. Cardio is great and we need it. Its the major exercise component to dropping the weight. However, cardio +strength is a dynamic duo that when done properly will assist you in the losing the weight and forming (sculpting) your body.

Make the commitment to incorporate strength training into your workout regimen and do it on alternate days of your cardio or lower impact exercises.

Strength training variations

You can do **Calisthenics** which are exercises that only rely on your body weight. These exercises are performed with different levels of intensity and rhythm. There are actually seven basic movements the human body can perform and all other exercises are merely variations of these seven: Pull, Push, Squat, Lunge, Hinge, Rotation and Gait. When doing all of these movements, you will be able to stimulate all of the major muscle groups in your body. So if you're choosing to do leg lifts, mountain climbers, push-ups, lunges, squats, burpees or even the superman exercise; they all originate from one of the seven basic exercise movements mentioned.

Another form of strength training is **Weight Lifting**. I'd like to clear up any misconceptions you've had in the past regarding lifting weights... weights are for girls too! Many women tend to shy away from weights because we are afraid we will have muscles popping out everywhere and we will look like men. Not so! I promise you.

Women that have the muscles popping out all over the place, look that way intentionally. They are considered body builders and train as well eat a certain way to get those results. So picking up 10 & 12lb dumbbells at the gym isn't going to bulk you up. There is also a tendency to feel awkward as a beginner with weight lifting; so as a newbie, I suggest reaching out for help.

If you choose to go to classes, most instructors incorporate the use of dumbbells and have a variety for all fitness levels. If you want to explore the weight room floor at the gym or lift weights at home, get help when starting out so that you are using proper form. In the wonderful world of the internet, you can watch videos at home to show you proper form if you don't have a trainer.

One of the greatest benefits for me when lifting and also from doing my girly push-ups; was starting to see my shoulders mold into this nice sleek sexy form. It was like the balls of my shoulders were no longer fat! The feeling I got when I picked something up - around the house and happen to notice my newly forming biceps was priceless! And push-ups became my go to body weight exercises when I began to see my collar bones again. When I was overweight, it's like I didn't realize that my collar bones, shoulders and biceps were covered in fat and there was a whole new world of sexiness underneath that fat! It's because we are so focused on the obvious; you know our breast, thighs, belly and the butt. So yes, you will feel some discomfort when lifting weights and sometimes you will feel like its too hard to do; but your body is screaming and reacting to something new. Don't fight it but welcome the new change, the new challenge into your routine. However, guided weight training until you are comfortable and confident is vital to properly incorporating strength training to avoid injury.

Helpful Workout Aids

Knowing your numbers - Just as we frequent the scale to see what that number is; we should invest in a good **heart rate monitor** to view your heart rate while working out. That number is really important! There were many years when I refused to wear one because I just didn't think it mattered much, or was necessary. The truth is, we are blindly working out if we don't know what our heart rate is. The heart-rate monitor lets you see if you are pushing hard enough during the walk, jog, run, or even during the HITT workouts. You want to insure you are giving it your all and recovering when you need to. The monitor also helps insure you are not over training; as over training can lead to injury. The overall goal is to be in your fat burning zone while exercising and then toning it down if you start to see that number on your monitor escalate too much. The beauty in this is that your numbers aren't the same as your spouses or friend's numbers. As you hit the fat burning zone, you will see results on the scale so give it your all during those workouts.

Not ready to hit the gym or hire a trainer? - But still need some direction - I've listed below some popular work our apps and videos that you can download or access on your smart phone. The convenience of theses apps allows you workout in your living room or the driveway if you choose.

FITON
Chloe-Ting (YouTube)
Skimble Workout Trainer
HITT Interval Training Timer
MadFit (YouTube)
Toni Mitchell (YouTube)
7 Minute Workout
JEFIT Workout Tracker
Nike Training Club
Runkeeper - GPS Track Run Walk

Working out after Injury

The loud impact to my car that I encountered while sitting in an intersection one day permanently affected the left side of my body. Initially, I did not think I was injured but after the adrenaline wore off, the truth was revealed. My neck and the entire left side of my body was in excruciating pain. The accident caused disc to rupture in my neck and lower back in several places. I sought treatment from Doctors and Chiropractors to begin the recovery process. The physical therapy appointments really benefited me as the goal was to regain strength and full range of motion in my legs. Never in my life had I thought I would encounter something like that. This accident also affected me mentally because I just felt bad. I didn't feel pretty with having to wear athletic walking shoes all the time; regardless to how nice my clothes looked. It caused me physical pain when I wore really flat shoes or shoes that were too high. For months I was inflamed and walked around in chronic pain. I also had constant headaches, and I just ate! This was a traumatic experience for me.

I couldn't workout and during that time I didn't see myself being able to workout for quite a while. My body needed to heal and I had to yield to the process mentally and physically. So boot camp classes and Orange Theory had to be put on hold. Eventually, I was finally able to begin working out but I needed to be wise about how I eased back into it. See this change to my body was so significant that I couldn't even clean my entire house in 1 day like I could before; needless to say, I wasn't ready to jump back into a 1-hour strenuous workouts.

As I eased my way back into workouts and making better food choices, I had to be sure and let to tell the trainer that I needed a revised version of certain exercises. Although my accident was a few years ago, I still practice wisdom when it comes to certain exercises that I am sure will aggravate the nerves in my back. For instance, superman exercises and routines that over extend my back are no longer a part of my regimen. There are plenty of modified or alternative exercises I can do that will give me the same results. I often do planks which give me a great core workout. It still disturbs me that I have very little balance on my left side to do lunges; but I don't avoid them. I just do them to the best of my ability and a little slower than everyone else around me. Since the accident, I still have to be sure that I properly stretch after exercising and I occasionally use a heating pad when necessary.

My point here is that although I had to pause from working out and allow my body to heal, I didn't give up. I didn't just give in and say I was never going to exercise again.

Although my experience was a bit drastic; the same principle applies if you were to strain, pull or experience a tear to a muscle while working out. Another way to cause injury to your muscles is to jump right into exercise without a pre -workout stretch. It's also important to stretch after your workouts regardless to how exhausted you may feel. Your body benefits greatly from stretching. There are several benefits from adopting a post workout stretch regimen.

Gains From Stretching:

Increased Flexibility
Improved Blood circulation
Eliminates Lactic Acid
Boost your energy
Pain Prevention
Improved Range of Motion
Increased Muscular Coordination
Slows the Body down (intense exercise can exhaust the body and cause one to feel drained)

Mental clarity and mind-body connection

Its also good to invest in a foam roller to assist you with post workout stretching. If your body has experienced a traumatic injury such as an accident of some sort, always seek medical advice from your physician and if you are healthy enough to strength train, please speak up and let your trainer know you need a modified version of certain exercises.

Winding It Down - Rest Days

Rest and recovery are essential in this journey and is just as important as exercise. As you plan your workout schedule, its important to include a couple of days to relax those muscles. Rest allows your muscles to rebuild and enables muscle growth. My current workouts usually consist of 3 days of cardio (5-6 mile walk). I often trade one of the walk days for a 30 minute HITT day. The remaining 2 days of the week I strength train (Orange Theory). So I desperately look forward to my 2 days of rest. However, I stagger the rest days... they aren't back-to-back. I usually rest on Sunday and Wednesday. There are several benefits to resting if you are really beating the pavement or putting the time in at the gym. Rest allows time for recovery, Prevents Muscle Fatigue, Reduces risk of injury, Improves Performance (on workout days), and Supports healthy sleep.

So although by now you may be rambunctious and ready to get the pounds off, you must find balance and allow your body to recover. As you rest physically, I also encourage you to rest mentally. Take some time to participate in your favorite hobby or enjoy a day to binge watch your favorite TV series. Do something you enjoy that does not require exerting a lot of energy. My favorite way to rest is to schedule a massage twice a month on a Sunday. The massage really works out the knots in my muscles and it helps me to decompress mentally. Taking time for rejuvenating physically and mentally benefits us in so many ways and I believe it makes us happier people in general.

"There is virtue in work and there is virtue in rest. Use both and overlook neither" Alan Cohen

Participation time:

In the space provided below:

Take a moment to list how you will begin your exercise regime. How will you incorporate exercise with fasting?

_____

_____

_____

_____

What's your favorite way to get moving and which days of the week will you commit to working out?

_____

_____

_____

_____

_____

10.

Divorce the Extras

PANCAKES AS BIG as the skillet! Yes! This was my go to breakfast; and pancakes made me feel good! On Saturday mornings I would getup and do my chores because I was looking forward to the nice nap I was going to take after eating the warm fluffy cake dripping with syrup and butter. The thick juicy polish sausage just completed the meal.

Growing up in a large family certain foods were a staple for us because it was cheap to prepare and was filling to the belly. So needless to say, we ate them almost weekly; alternating with grits and biscuits on the following Saturday. My mom seemed to have an art for making these large cakes and she knew just when to flip them so they didn't fold or break while cooking. I loved them as a child and my love for them continued into adulthood. Breakfast just wasn't breakfast without a pancake and warm coffee and maybe even a side of eggs. I made them often for my family and I even got a little fancy by adding orange extract to my batter and they loved it!

As I got serious about my weight loss, this was actually a pleasure I had to divorce.

The sluggish feeling I felt all day from the heavy pancakes not to mention the scale tipping in the wrong direction was just counter productive to my progress.

Yes when we're not fasting, we can eat what we choose in our feeding window... but this just wasn't working for me.

I found myself trying to out-exercise the plate of pancakes.

This was also the same for me regarding oatmeal. Growing up Dad made the best oatmeal in the world; and I had learned to make it the same way.

It wasn't the instant stuff! It was Quaker Oats in the tall box with the round top and it had to be cooked on the stove. Dad loaded it with brown sugar, cinnamon, butter and occasionally raisins. In the winter months he would pour a little cold milk over the plate of oatmeal and it would cool off the hot cereal so we could quickly eat before school.

I took that tradition to my children and in my early years of weight loss attempts, I would have a big bowl after leaving the gym in the mornings. I simply just didn't know any better.

I felt that since it was oats, it was healthy and nutritious for me; however the added sugar and butter made it high in fat. As much as I loved oatmeal, I decided to part with it all together because making healthier versions just wasn't appealing to my taste buds... so I have been better off without it.

The rich sweet taste of doughnuts are also a memory of the past for me. They simply just contain too much sugar and quickly spike my insulin.

Another favorite I had to part with was nuts - believe it or not; particularly almonds.

Yes, almonds are good for us (raw almonds) but because I could not eat just a few, you know just 1 serving. I had to let them go! See, I wouldn't just eat 1 or 2 servings, I would find myself eating the entire can in one day! This was the case because I was eating roasted and heavily salted almonds. It was just something about the salt and crunchy texture that just kept me wanting more!

In recent years, the manufacturer of the brand I like so much introduced hot and spicy ones, barbecue and my favorite salt and vinegar!

Yep, salt and vinegar almonds!

I had to make a decision to part ways with these foods that I seemed to over indulged in. Foods that I just seem to lose my mind over! Foods that I couldn't seem to control the need to keep eating after just a few bites.

So I had to write up the divorce decree. I made the decision not to eat them any more and now passing them on the grocery store isle is not a problem.

Since I have adapted a fasting lifestyle, I can even prepare pancakes for my husband without participating. See, I can enjoy pancakes, oatmeal, doughnuts or salt and vinegar almonds in my eating window but I choose not to because I'd rather eat food that will give me energy vs making me feel sluggish.

The Crave - Is it keeping us Fat?

So why is it that we crave certain foods and just cant seem to get enough of them? Why is it that a little is not enough and we eat the entire bag of chips vs just a serving?

Why can't we seem to pass up the doughnuts at the gas station when we're running in for coffee?

Why are we addicted to the soda, cookies and deep fried food?

I'll tell you why - See we as consumers have been heavily studied at least since the mid to late 1960's. Food manufacturers hire consultants and consumer scientist to identify our emotional needs and target them with preciseness. The large sales of processed foods in our country can be attributed to the research done on us as consumers. Consumer scientist have even conducted experiments in which they placed devices on the heads of shoppers to track their eye movements as they roam the store, and the results from this tracking helped to define where products are placed on the shelves in supermarkets. For instance, products placed at eye level on the shelf are considered the prime spot. However, the special displays or end caps at the end of an isle are actually more profitable than the eye level spots on shelves. Food manufactures compete for these spots on grocery store shelves to get us to buy their products and to make their pockets bigger! But let's explore a deeper reason as to why we crave the processed foods that keep us desiring Salt, Sugar and Fat. A Precious Jewel to the processed food industry over the years has been a man by the name of Howard Moskowitz. Moskowitz was a student at Harvard and he decided to do his thesis on human taste.

During this time, so little was known about why people like the foods they do and he focused on creating a scientific method by which researchers could study taste. He would experiment with mixtures of sweet with salty, salty with bitter, and bitter with other flavors. He conducted these studies on campus with fellow students and he would pay them fifty cents to tell him which ones they liked and which ones they did not. His goal was to rework food. This was done by playing with the magical formula of salt, sugar and fat. For more than thirty years he has worked behind the scenes to rescue many companies that had decreased sales in the processed food industry. As he perfected his craft over the years some of his biggest clients were Dr. Pepper, Campbell Soup, General Foods, Kraft and Pepsi Co.

The experiments he conducted using high math and computations had one goal in mind - to **Create The Biggest Crave**. His ability to create the biggest crave in consumers is termed as the **"Bliss Point"**. He would search for just the right amount of certain ingredients to generate the greatest appeal among consumers. This process took intense study and research because too little of this, or too much of that might ruin a products taste or texture and negative results would affect a manufacture's sales. In the language of product developers this is known as **optimization**. In an interview with Michael Moss the author of Salt, Sugar, Fat; Mokowitz is not bashful in saying that he has been a game changer with many products. He mentions being successful with optimizing pizzas, salad dressings and pickles; just to mention a few. And to be clear here, he was not necessarily inventing new products but taking existing products using his high math and computations, and **engineering** them. Therefore, being able to create the **Biggest Crave**. So… you're not alone… and there is nothing wrong with you when you find yourself craving the popular prepackaged foods that contain high amounts of salt, sugar and fat. There has been much work put into us craving the chocolate, pizza or the chips.

I want to assure you here that as you become a more experienced faster and especially as you begin to implement longer hours of fasting, you will crave the junk food less. You will be able to walk down the grocery store isles without the doughnuts and chips calling your name like they used to.

I have personally found that fasting crushes the cravings that kept me fat for many years. This really began to happen for me as I used the **OMAD AND ADF** methods of fasting. Fasting became a new discipline in my life that has forever changed when and how I eat. See-when you focus on the 1 to 2 meals per day and focus on your feeding window you will find you won't have much room for the junk food. Consuming foods that will sustain you won't have you thinking about the junk anymore. Trust me…its true!

Parting Ways-

In addition to me divorcing the foods mentioned, I also had to at least curtail when and how much I ate certain foods. For me those food choices are wheat, grains, potatoes and most dairy products.

Now don't freak out on me! I'm not saying that I don't eat them at all… I have just leaned to limit my intake of them. See while we are working to drop the pounds through fasting and working out, we also need to be concerned about reducing inflammation in our bodies. And for me - greatly reducing the intake of wheat, dairy and grains and potatoes works for me. For example, I may have r bread with my meal or cake for dessert, but not often.

When dining out occasionally I may order some rice with my meal. These are foods that personally don't give me energy; so I choose not to eat them on a regular basis. Pasta such as spaghetti, fettuccine and lasagna are a memory of the past as well. I just feel too heavy, bloated and sluggish after eating these foods. On the contrary, I do splurge on Mac & Cheese on holidays or special occasions. Yep it's a culture thing...

The intent of this chapter is not to instruct or suggest that you never eat another slice of pie, or enjoy pasta, chocolate or potato chips; but to simply to bring awareness and to get you to thinking of the extras that you may be indulging in (too often) that could be hindering your progress.

I invite you to make this personal. Evaluate what your vices are when it comes to certain foods. Maybe you're putting too much cream and sugar in your coffee in the morning? If your cup of coffee is light-skinned or white - we have a problem! You may find it necessary to make the switch to black coffee if you can handle it or reduce the amount of cream and sugar you add to your coffee. Personally, I don't preach much about coffee intake because although I fast every day, I am considered a "dirty faster" because I do enjoy cream in my coffee every morning. Its the one luxury I never gave up but was still able to lose weight.

One a side note, I was talking with a friend one day some years ago as she was in a drive thru ordering breakfast. I heard her order a large coffee and twelve packets of sugar. Yes twelve packets! I was stunned! I absolutely could not believe one could consume so much sugar in a cup of coffee.

Or maybe your salads aren't as healthy as they could be and you're scratching your head as to why you're not seeing the results you want. Are you still drowning your salads with dressings that are higher in fat or sugar? Are your salads loaded with cheese, processed deli meats and croutons to make you feel better about eating salad?

Just maybe its time to consider and explore less fattening salad dressings or make your own. There are countless recipes for making a healthier salad dressing online. My personal favorite dressing to make is apple cider vinegar dressing. Another culprit could be that you're eating too much cheese. I recently heard a young lady say" I love cheese, I eat a lot of it because I thought it was healthy for me".

While cheese is a good source of fat for us, over indulging can be counter productive to your results.

Could your problem be with condiments? Or consuming too much of them? Are you a lover of mayo and like to load up on the sauces at restaurants?

You know what your weaknesses and triggers are so it's time to decide what you need to divorce, separate or take a break from so you can start to see greater results.

This isn't much different from ending a bad relationship with a person. After many months or years of being in a dysfunctional or toxic relationship, you finally woke up to the fact that you needed to end it because it was no longer mentally or physically healthy for you. The same goes for many foods that have given you temporary pleasure for the moment but have left you physically sick!

As I write this chapter, I am thinking of a young lady that is 29 years old and is currently in the hospital after having a stroke. We don't know if she is going to make it out because the conditions are bad. My dear friends… we have got to begin to break up with some of these habitual food choices that are leading to heart attacks, strokes kidney disease and more! **Love yourself enough to fight for you!**

A closer look-

Maybe the extra's in your diet don't involve food and you are choosing to **Drink Your Calories** more so than eating them. I have a couple of friends that love Pepsi or Sweet Tea. The one that loves Pepsi, prefers it over food. She could go many hours throughout the day and not pick up a piece of food but when trying to remember how many cans of Pepsi she had consumed that day she couldn't tell you. As soon she decided to curtail her soda intake, the pounds began to fall off. The friend that loves the sweet tea is still a work in progress; but I just love her to life and often encourage her to drink more water throughout the day. What we have to consider when it comes to drinking our calories is that many beverages can have the caloric intake of a meal or a small snack and If you're still going to have lunch or dinner in your eating window; you may want to reconsider your caloric intake from beverages.

For instance, many of the specialty coffee drinks that we tend to buy that come with floating whipped cream on top can average from 200-300 calories. Another precaution to take when drinking your calories is that liquid calories don't help you feel full. Something else to consider when drinking your calories is that sweetened beverages are quickly absorbed in the body. As a result, our insulin needs to respond quickly in an effort to keep our blood sugar in control. Regular consumption of sugary drinks wears out our insulin and we become insulin resistant.

Some additional behaviors that maybe hindering your progress can be **Eating While Cooking -** At times we can develop this terrible habit of constantly tasting and sampling the dishes we are preparing for the family. I know for me in the earlier years this is usually when I am making macaroni and cheese for the family dinner. I would have the tendency to keep tasting it to be sure it was salted enough or to be sure the cheeses were blended just right with the butter. Macaroni and cheese is something most people make according to eye measurement and we just add the milk, cheese, butter... until it tastes right before baking in the oven. I had to learn to actually write my recipe down once I got it the way I liked it. Subsequently, I just followed my own recipe which eliminated the need for tasting while cooking. Let's face it, the calories can add up pretty quickly, and we really need to be mindful so we aren't sabotaging our progress.

Mindless Eating - Snacking when you're not hungry - You will find that this journey of fasting can and will be challenging. Fasting is definitely an act of discipline. And I get it... that delaying eating your favorite foods is something you've never done before in your life. However, I promise you as you follow the plan, create the eating and fasting window that works best for you... the results will follow!

Slip-ups-

Personally, during my slip-up moments; I would find myself eating my husband's chips at 8:30pm when I was supposed to be fasting. I had to quickly correct that behavior because I didn't want to start the pattern of making excuses for myself. See this was when I was a little over half way to my goal. I was thirty five pounds down and people were noticing my progress. And yes, I was feeling good about myself! However, as I mentioned earlier... sometimes we fail because we become too comfortable with the progress we've made and we start to revert backwards.

I also encourage you to evaluate why you're picking up the snack? Are you stressed about something? Are you bored? When I really got serious about the results I wanted, I had to ignore the snacks in my house that belonged to my family members because we didn't have the same goals in mind.

So, as you begin the journey, decide you are going to discipline yourself to only eat in your feeding window. Will you have slip-ups sometimes? Sure, because you're human; however too many slips-ups and too often will show up on the scale and in your clothes.

Eating the kids left overs - Many of us don't like to waste food and we grew up that way because maybe food was hard to come by. Maybe your parents trained you to eat everything on your plate. Who remembers sitting in the chair crying because you wanted to get up from the dinner table? You sat there and cringed at your Mom or Dad's voice that said you're not getting up until you finish the liver or sweet peas! Because of this many of us have trained ourselves over the years to clean the plate. Now that we have children, we have carried that same principle to our own households. Except- we maybe realizing that our children are a bit more strong-willed today than we were growing up. So we allow them to get up and leave the table before their plate is clean. Keeping that mindset - often results with us eating the scraps of chicken or bread from our children's plates so we aren't wasting food. How about making smaller plates for the kids so they will finish their meals? This alleviates the guilt you may feel for throwing out food.

Eating too many calories in your feeding window - When we are fasting especially in the early days of starting out, we are so famished... we envision eating the entire kitchen when our feeding window opens! I especially felt this way when I was doing OMAD on a particular day. I had waited 23 hours to eat and I wanted it all! When first starting OMAD, I would usually do it on the weekends when I wasn't working. I usually ate out on the days I was having the meal. However, I would often find that I was over doing it. I would order a meal from a restaurant and I would sometimes order dessert and lemonade. The problem with me doing this was that I wasn't always listening to my body. See you will find that your stomach is shrinking as you continue in this fasting lifestyle. I often found I really couldn't eat all of the food that I ordered and I was in fact full about half way through the meal. But because my mindset had not totally shifted in the right direction, I would keep eating. I would finish the meal and the dessert. As a result, if I decided to weigh myself the next morning - you can imagine what I saw... yes an increased number.

Just to clarify - I was never a scale addict in my process but I used the scale often to gauge my progress. I wanted to know how certain foods affected my body especially on days that I did not workout. So I want you to be mindful of how much food you 're consuming during your feeding window. Regardless to if you have chosen to count calories in your process or not. Even if you don't count calories, listen to your body. Stop eating when you are full. Not stuffed! So when you honestly know you have had enough... push the plate away. Trust me as you begin to practice this discipline, you will be rewarded when you try on that fabulous outfit!

This brings me to my next point regarding cheat days. There are many opinions out there regarding cheat days or cheat meals and ultimately you will have to decide what works for you. However, I will say that its easier to recover from one high caloric meal vs an entire "cheat day".

Stick with your plan, stick with what works for you to continue to see the progress you've gained. But also take some time to enjoy life.

Sometimes you will eat the cookie or slice of cake but be mindful in how often you indulge.

If indulgence takes you into a week or two of binge eating - its time to reassess your goals. Its time to remember your Why.

"Don't exchange what you want most for what you want at the moment" Uknown

Participation time:

In the space provided below:

Take a few moments to identify which foods or areas that you need to divorce or separate from so you aren't sabotaging your progress. Once you have identified them, record the changes you will actually make.

_____

_____

_____

_____

_____

_____

_____

_____

11.

Crushing Intimidation

STANDING IN FRONT of the weight machine acting as if I was tying my shoe lace or pretending to adjust my clothing was something I found myself doing (in the early years of working out); when I was really just trying to figure out how to use the equipment.

I'd even secretly watch other people use a machine so I didn't look like a fool when I attempted to use it. I even remember walking out of a workout class one day because a series of mishaps during that class just made me want to quit! For starters, my butt has slipped off the water rowing machine because I was learning how to use it. So of course, I felt stupid and it was obvious to others around me that I was a beginner. I also had an encounter with the TRX bands in class that day - I didn't know how to use them. Although the instructor demoed the alligator arm exercise and the exercise movement was on the display screen above my head, I just couldn't seem to get it… by the time I got it halfway figured out, it was time to move on to the next exercise. The final straw for me that day was when we moved over to the weight room floor, I was surrounded by a group of bulky men and over achieving athletic women in a small space. I felt closed in and intimidated; so I grabbed my water bottle and towel and just left! I left that day holding in my tears with the intention to cancel my membership.

I just didn't feel like I belonged there... and besides, I had never spent that much money on a monthly membership to anyplace in my entire life!

The Embarrassment

I think my most embarrassing moment (in my YMCA days) was when I took a step aerobics class and I looked like I had two left feet! I actually faked as if I hurt my ankle to give me an excuse to leave. I attended this class with a friend that loved to dance and was an extreme zumba lover. So I thought I'd give it a try. I guess you've figured out by now that I'm not very coordinated and its true that surely - I can't dance! So you will never find me in a zumba, step aerobics or hip-hop dance class trying to burn some calories. Remember - I grew up in a preacher's house so dancing has never been my thing. I wasn't allowed to go to parties and we couldn't even play secular music in the house; so where was I supposed to get this rhythm from to participate in zumba or hip-hop dance classes?

So although I walked out of class that day feeling clumsy, feeling low, feeling intimated I didn't quit. I showed up for my next scheduled class. See I had to go home and talk to myself. I had to encourage myself to shake it off and to go back. I had to give myself a break. "Faith... you're just starting, there will be new experiences and although they will be challenging, you have to show up again." See I knew that in the long run, these workouts would be good for my body, they would transform my body, they would make me stronger physically. So I had to keep going.

I just had to come to the realization that certain classes or forms of exercise weren't for me. I've learned to embrace what I can do and show up! I'm all about the boot camps, toning classes, hill running on treadmills, weight lifting (within my means), water rowing (now that I can operate it); as well as walking and running outside in the fresh air.

I've shared my embarrassing and truthful experiences with you because I want you to know that I had to refuse to be intimated and so do you. I'd like to share with you some tips on crushing intimidation in this journey. This can relate to a few areas as you walk this thing out. There can be a tendency to feel intimidated when it comes to working out, when we are learning to fast and even when it comes to our wardrobe as your weight changes. Although we may face intimidation; one thing I know for sure is that we can Crush it!

See intimation stems from fear- Maybe its fear of not knowing what to do and looking stupid in the eyes of others, maybe the entire process feels a little overwhelming and you're afraid of failing. Maybe you're afraid of starting because you don't know what you're going to look like when you're finished; when you've met your goal. Maybe you're afraid of change - because you don't know what life will look like on the other side of change. I had a friend to tell me once (that had made some significant weight loss progress) that she wanted to stop in the middle of her journey because she was afraid of what she was going to look like skinny. She was afraid of looking sickly, having a lot of lose skin and how others would view her appearance. She had been overweight as a child and had never seen a skinny version of herself.

So how do we crush it? How do we crush feeling intimidated in this process; regardless to how the intimidation comes?

Ask for help-

After wiping the tears from my awful experience that day in class - I had to decide I was going back to class and handle business. First I had to internally acknowledge I didn't know what I was doing. I also had to verbalize that I needed help. So I showed up for the next class and stayed after to ask the instructor questions. She was more than willing to go over using proper form for the exercises we went over in class. I also noticed, the more I showed up… some of the high achievers in class would often give an encouraging word if I was struggling next to them. So it's time to let go of the fear and shame of not knowing and ask questions.

This is also true when it comes to Fasting. Yes... This is new to you and you may not even be sure yet that you want to stick this out. So I encourage you to ask for help in the fasting groups on line or research problems you may encounter as you go. You can also refer back to the fasting chapter in this book if you feel stuck or need more direction. The point I'm trying to make here is that no question is too small or too simple to ask.

As I made progress towards my goal, I noticed that my right eye started to twitch or spasm for a few weeks. I knew it was related to my food intake but I just didn't know how it was related.

So I did some research online and received help from a couple fasting experts and my question was completely answered. What I discovered after switching to OMAD for approximately three weeks, is that I was having the symptom because my body was lacking electrolytes. I needed to be sure I was continuing to open my eating window with bone broth and I added a couple of supplements into my diet. One in particular was a magnesium supplement. The twitching of the eye went away after a couple of weeks as my body came back into balance by taking in the proper nutrients.

Don't worry about what others think-

As you navigate through fasting and working out you will get a plunder of opinions and expressed thoughts from those you love. The family and friends that don't have weight loss issues will give you their opinions. The friends that have successfully lost the weight will tell you what you're doing wrong. They will try to convince you that you're harming yourself by going without food for so many hours. The friends that want you to remain fat will tell you – you're just doing the most! Just doing too much! Or my favorite from a friend was…" Please don't lose any more weight, don't get too skinny… we don't want you looking like a drug addict".

If you listen to the negative opinions of others, you won't get anywhere! I encourage you to do as little talking as necessary about your fasting and working out until you are comfortable and confident with the process. As you start to see results and its obvious to others as well, you may be a little more comfortable with sharing what you are doing to lose the weight.

Personally, I sort of went into hiding for several months when I started fasting. The feeling of wanting to crawl under one of the tables at my mom's birthday party because I was the heaviest I had ever been; is something I would never forget and never wanted to revisit. I left there with the determination to finally lose the weight. However, I was quiet about my internal desire for change. I didn't really know how I was going to do but I was tired of failing. Something something had to change! I even waited a month or so before revealing to my husband that I was fasting because I wanted to be sure it was working for me. He had always been supportive of me throughout our relationship with any life goal I had, but he's not a fan of fasting. And I was OK with that. I had to do what was best for me and what worked for me. Although the voices and influence of your family really matter, your self care has to become priority. Its an individual walk. I became comfortable with my fasting community and just put the work in behind the scenes. Eventually when I did go to see family and friends it was 6 months in to my journey and I was 28lbs down. When asked; I still did not reveal the details of my journey. My programmed response was "girl, I'm just putting the work in!"

Dismiss the chatter in your own head-

Aside from the opinions of others, you also have to dismiss the negative chatter in your own head. You know those thoughts that come up to remind you of how many times you failed before when trying to lose weight. Those thoughts of "you're not gonna make it this time either". I want you to assure you that you're going to succeed this time! You are significant, you matter and you are enough! You can do this but you have to get started and fight to keep going! You will meet your goal weight and live a healthier life.

Be Assertive-

Crushing intimidation requires assertiveness. Being assertive is about being your own proponent (advocate) for yourself. When it comes to working out, look the part! Show up as if you are ready. Show up as if you are just as important as everyone else there.

Invest in some decent workout clothes within your budget. If you're a girly-girl like me; color coordinate those workout clothes and look cute while you sweat it out! A good quality running shoe is essential. Even if you are not a runner and you're more of a walker, purchasing a running show will insure you have good stability and avoid foot pain. Personally, I wear Nike Running Shoes and occasionally wear a man's running shoe in different brands. Generally, when wearing a man's running shoe, you will go down a size or two from your normal size. Also, lets not forget to protect the girls! Purchase a good sports bra or two to keep the girls lifted and to keep you confident while working out.

Regardless to what the number reads on your scale; don't allow people, equipment, or environments to intimidate you!

"Nobody can make you feel inferior without your consent" Eleanor Roosevelt

Self Affirmation Crushes Intimidation-

There will be times when you feel low or less than when learning a new workout, facing a new challenge while fasting ;or even when you are working out next to the super athletic person in the gym. But I'd like to encourage you to talk yourself out of those feelings. We can't wait for someone to encourage us or to pull us out of an emotional slump. You've got to square your shoulders and talk to yourself! When you feel like quitting or have that feeling of what's the use!... reverse it with" I'm becoming stronger and fitter every day", I love and care for my body", "I am running my own race regardless to what others say or do, "I enjoy training", "Fasting cleans my body of all toxins", "Hour by hour I am getting happier, healthier and clearer as my body cleanses itself, I am reclaiming my health and well-being".

At one point in my process, I was doing some grocery shopping one day and it just seemed as if I was just honing in on little petite women as I shopped for my food. I started to feel low and a little depressed as I admired their tiny waistlines. At that time I was 35 pounds lighter and it had been at least 10 years since I was in the 170's on the scale. I had to talk myself out of feeling down although I could still see a stomach roll and my breast size didn't seem to be reducing fast enough. I had to choose to change my perspective about my progress. I decided to go home and try on the clothing that I still owned that were too big to remind myself of how far I had come. I also took some time to coordinate outfits in my new size and just chose to love & accept myself - right where I was in the journey. Not to focus on the 50lb goal; but to enjoy the now. We've got to crush the low moments with positive thoughts and words about ourselves to gain the fortitude to keep going.

"If you spend all your time thinking about how someone is going to one-up you, you can't put your best foot forward" Miranda Kenneally

Participation time:

In the space provided below:

How or in what areas have you felt intimidation when it comes to weight loss?

_____

_____

_____

_____

_____

Do you now believe you can crush it?
What's your plan? How will you stand up to intimidation?

_____

_____

_____

_____

_____

12.

Digging Deeper

UGGH! I WAS stuck at 168 pounds and feeling low. I was following my normal fasting regimen and workouts but I just seemed to be stuck… I had hit a plateau again. My progress seem to come to a halt.

It's common and if you haven't experienced it yet, - you will. As explained earlier, a plateau simply means you haven't gained any weight but you haven't lost any either. "You may notice when starting out within the first few weeks or even the first couple of months that you are able to drop weight at a rapid pace.

Lets examine this scientifically: This is because when you cut calories the body gets needed energy initially by releasing its stores of glycogen, a type of carbohydrate found in the muscles and liver.

Glycogen is partly made of water, so when glycogen is burned for energy, it releases water, resulting in weight loss that's mostly water. This effect is temporary, however as you lose weight, you lose some muscle along with fat.

Muscle helps keep the rate at which you burn calories (metabolism) up. So as you lose weight, your metabolism declines, causing you to burn fewer calories than you did at your heavier weight.

Your slower metabolism will slow your weight loss, even if you eat the same number of calories or same amount of food that helped you lose weight. When the calories you burn equal the calories you eat, you reach a plateau.

So, If you've found that your progress is stagnate. It's time to evaluate where and how some changes can be made to break through the plateau. When you've stalled, it can get you down a little and you may doubt the process; but I want to encourage you not to give up but suggest that maybe it's time to **Dig Deeper**.

Embrace the small changes

At a particular point in my process; my goal that month was to get to 163 by the end of the month. The goal was to move from 168 to 163. However, I just couldn't understand why the scale wasn't moving and it frustrated me! On one particular after noon while thinking about my progress I happened to receive a package delivery. It was a jumpsuit that I had forgotten that I ordered. After working, I rushed to try it on and to my surprise it fit great. I had never been able to bring myself to purchase jumpsuits when I was 200 or even 180 pounds.

I hated the way I looked in them. Because my belly was as big as my butt, I just felt like I resembled a round glazed doughnut or like a woman wearing a tire. I just felt awful while in dressing rooms trying on jumpers.

However, my new jumper was black and had flared sleeves and my waistline was snatched in this outfit! I looked and felt amazing. Trying the outfit on that afternoon took my focus off of being stuck at 168. It took my focus away from wishing I weighed less. I must have worn the outfit for about an hour in the house that day. I pranced in the mirror and tried it on with different shoes. I couldn't resist looking at myself and admiring my defined waist-line. My Fupa was finally shrinking!; and it was really noticeable.

I also decided to take my measurements that day and realized I had gone from a size 38DDD to 38D in bra size. I had also lost 14 inches overall in my belly, breast and thigh areas from when I started. My clothing size at that point was a size 10 jeans (although a little snug). I had to stop and realize the size 10 jeans that were a little snug was a great achievement over the size 16/18 jeans when I started my journey.

What I realized that day was that sometimes we have to dig deeper within when we are feeling low or defeated. We have to remember the **WHY**. We have to remind ourselves of why we have started this fasting lifestyle. We have to remind ourselves of how far we have come even if we aren't where we want to be. Remind yourself of how your habits have changed from picking up the cookies to selecting a nice firm apple. Remind yourself of how many days you have chosen to get off the couch and hit the gym. Remind yourself of how your blood pressure or blood sugar levels have improved since you started. Once you've been able to recall your accomplishments, this will give you the boost you need to keep going. It will take your focus off the number on the scale. I simply needed to be reminded that I had not seen 160's range on the scale in 20 years or so. So I needed to just enjoy the moment. My dear friends… this is an opportunity to focus on being grateful for the process of Now… to embrace where you are now and enjoy it.

We must like and love ourselves - If no one else in the world does… you have to become comfortable with YOU… and give yourself permission to love you! The practice of Self-Love is essential on a regular basis in this journey of weight loss. As a matter of fact, because life can be so hard and cruel; I believe its necessary on a daily basis to practice self-love.

What do I mean by self-love? First, let me clarify that self-love isn't being obsessed with yourself or so self-consumed that no one can stand to be around you. Rather… self-love is defined as:

having a high regard for your own well-being and happiness. It means taking care of your own needs and not sacrificing your well-being to please others.

So here is what it looks like to practice self-love on a regular basis:

Speak kind words to and about yourself daily -

"Girl, you are gorgeous"! "I am fearfully and wonderfully made". "I am a unique individual and there is no one else in the world like me", "I look great, feel great and there is nothing anyone can do about it"!

Choose to be positive- Practice thinking positive thoughts throughout the day even if it's difficult. We have to retrain our thoughts from dwelling on the negative side of a situation or circumstance. I must mention here that in the beginning chapters of the book when I described how I felt about my appearance; my thinking changed. As I progressed I had to practice self love and to speak positively about my image and my progress even if I didn't always feel it. We also need to choose positive environments. If you are dining with family, friends or even co-workers that are only spewing negativity about your fasting life style; kindly dismiss yourself from those environments. The work you are putting in is hard enough without having to deal with doubting Thomas and negative Nancy about how you are trying to improve your life. You owe no one an explanation for what you are doing and you have to love yourself enough to be your own cheerleader when necessary. Isn't it interesting how they had nothing to say when you were over weight, could barely walk and a slave to medications?

Fuel your body- Choose to fuel your body everyday with good food and drink in your eating window that will keep you nourished and energized. I made it a practice daily not to eat in a hurry. Since my eating window usually ranged within a 4-hour window; or just the 1-hour if I was doing OMAD - I never rushed to eat. I would plan ahead of what I was going to eat and I would choose a nice plate and glass - and enjoy my meal. I would sit at the table without distractions and enjoy it. See I had been thinking about that meal for many hours and I didn't want to be walking around, multi-tasking, talking on the phone or even scrolling social media when I enjoyed my 1 or 2 meals each day. This was hard for me to do at first, but it became easier as I viewed it as a way to love myself.

Celebrate You- I recall scheduling a date with my girlfriends whom I had not physically seen in over a year and I had not told them I was fasting. Before my date with them, I decided to buy a pair of jeans that actually fit. I picked three sizes and took them to the dressing room. The sizes were 14, 12 and 10. I actually didn't even try on the 14's because I knew they were too big. I tried on the 12's and they looked amazing on me. I took a chance and tried on the size 10 and I actually got them on and could button them! However... I did have a muffin top while wearing the 10's and decided to leave them at the store. But I just knew I was only a month or two away from fitting the 10's without the muffin top issue, so I was willing to be patient. So of course, I went to brunch looking great in my clothes; did my make-up that day and had a great time. My friends did complement my new size and I was grateful; but honestly my self-confidence was so high that day. I didn't need any compliments from anyone. I knew I looked good and felt good physically in my body! I felt strong and vibrant and just ready to take on the world that day. The atmosphere and the food during brunch made me feel like royalty! I enjoyed prime rib, shrimp, hummus, a variety of fruit & cheese and just really great food as I enjoyed the company of my friends. So I want to encourage you to treat yourself while you're in this process. It's OK to buy the pair of jeans (even if you haven't met your goal weight), buy yourself the bouquet of roses and put them on display just as you would if you had received them as a gift. Its far time for you to be happy being you!

Additional Ways To Dig Deeper

Aside from digging deeper emotionally and mentally when your progress stalls. You will find it necessary to **dig deeper** with your **workouts** or possibly adapt a **longer fasting period**.

When the body gets used to a certain routine, it becomes comfortable with what you're doing. Its like your body can predict... OK... she's gonna just walk 30 minutes three days a week and eat the same meals. As a result, the body decide to relax, chill and become accustom to what you've been doing. Consider working out a little longer. If you attend 30 minute classes, maybe it's time to do 45-to-60-minute classes.

One way I changed it up or tricked my body was when I agreed to go on a 8 mile hike with my sisters. I had never gone hiking before and it was a little tough. We got a little lost but enjoyed the overall experience. I burned 893 calories on that hike. So hiking is a way I chose to dig deeper for better results when I felt my progress was moving slow. I would also occasionally go for an 8 mile walk in my neighborhood.

Another suggestion is to try stair walking or running as opposed to just walking outside or on the treadmill. Search for stairs at an office complex that you could use after hours as a workout station. Stair workouts will definitely break your plateau! Trust me, I know from personal experience. Stair running makes you feel like you're going to die; but if you can stick with it, you are sure to see results. As workouts become tough, tell yourself to keep pushing! When you are coming to the end of your walk or run and want to give up; turn up the music in your headphones and drive harder! Walk or run faster to the finish line. I can recall one of my trainer's over the years that would say" come on Faith, give me eight more". That meant I had to push myself when I thought the workout was over and do the eight extra sets of what ever she was having me do.

When you don't change up your workout routine or fasting window for extended periods of time; you will notice the scale doesn't budge and you begin to feel stuck. We like to call it tricking the body - its what you have to do to shake things up and get the scale to moving in the right direction again. If you're feeling like you're stuck, take it to the next level and fast for longer periods of time. If you have been a stickler for 16:8; try adding on an extra 2 to 3 hours of fasting time. If you have never tried OMAD; definitely be willing to explore it for a least a few weeks so that your body breaks through the stagnation of the same routine.

I hope you're understanding here that you must find balance in this process. Its not always going to be a perfect journey and you will need to make adjustments along the way but if you stick with, you'll get the results you're looking for.

My first experience with a long fast was a 30-hour one and that happened by accident. I had a hair braiding appointment that lasted a lot longer than I anticipated. I arrived at the appointment while in my fasting window and assumed the stylist would be done with my hair by the time my eating window opened. I was sadly disappointed and needless to say, I became HANGRY! I eventually ate at the 30-hour mark and was content. Surprisingly, the next day I had dropped two pounds because of the longer fasting period. This also taught me that I could go longer. In just a few months after this experience, I ventured into longer fast more specifically ADF because I needed to simply go deeper; to push myself past my normal routine to see better results.

Something else to consider believe it or not is to evaluate your food intake to see if you're eating enough food. If you aren't eating enough, your body will hold on to your stored fat. Therefore, you don't see the scale move. Although I am not a fan of counting calories and seldom paid attention to counting; sometimes it's necessary to count or gauge your calorie intake to be sure you are fueling your body enough. I did occasionally find myself in that situation. Strangely enough what usually cures that is to eat a little more fat (healthy fat) or a little junk food (don't over do it). This will usually cause a little drop in your weight. I would grab a small bag of chips or a piece of cake. Again sometimes its about tricking the body; mixing things up to get the scale moving again. Suggesting a little junk food maybe surprising to read but if you think this lifestyle change is about eating the same boring salad every day to lose weight and to keep dropping the pounds, I would have to say that's "fake news". The driving point here is that you know when and decide how you need to dig deeper when your progress slows, stalls or gets a little discouraging along the way.

"Dig deep and empower yourself today. Stand in your inner strength. Be uniquely you" Amy Leigh-McCree

Participation time:

In the space provided below:

I invite you to do a self-inventory. How you can dig deeper to catapult your weight loss at this point in your journey?

_____

_____

_____

_____

_____

_____

_____

_____

_____

13.

Avoiding Relapse

MY SENSES WERE high and I was craving it! Lying in bed on a Sunday morning...

I could mentally visualize the sweet creamy- cream cheese icing that was neatly swirled over the moist dense carrot cupcake I had baked the day before. All I could think about was how good they were, how happy they made me feel and I wanted another one! Because cake (especially a moist cake) had been one of my closes friends over the years it just made me think happy thoughts as I chewed every piece. Scientifically, what happens in the brain when we eat the most calorie dense foods (that are high in fat), is a rewarding process. Our brains are rewarding our bodies with small burst of dopamine.

Dopamine is known as the feel-good neurotransmitter. The brain releases it when we eat food that we crave or while we have sex, contributing to feelings of pleasure and satisfaction as part of the reward system.

I was in my fasting window and I couldn't believe I was craving cake at 8:00am! See, I decided to splurge the day before because we had friends over for dinner. I chose to do OMAD that day because I had cooked a large soul-food meal for my husband and friends and I wanted to enjoy the food too!

I chewed slowly and savored every bite of the meal which consisted of: corn beef brisket, rice & peas, macaroni & cheese, charred brussels sprouts, grilled chicken; and for dessert, my succulent carrot cupcakes. I know it sounds like a lot of food , and it was. However, I was cautious with my portion sizes on the plate and I only ate half of my cupcake. See by this point I wasn't as afraid of the scale moving up a little (because my weight would stabilize the next day); more so than I was of having a belly ache all night from over eating.

The longer I laid in bed that morning, the more I thought about eating a cupcake. I was having an internal fight of whether I should continue to fast until my feeding window opened or if I was going to give in to the cupcake.

I decided to get up and clean the house and as I cleaned I still battled with the cupcake in my head and it even seem to be invading my taste buds! (Yes… the **Biggest Crave** effect)

As I was cleaning, I began to talk to myself (you know in my head). I thought about the consequences of breaking my fast and eating the cupcake. Eating the cupcake as my first meal would definitely spike my insulin levels, end my fast early and just make me feel awful.

In addition to feeling bad after eating it - I knew it would just send me into a spiral of bad eating for the entire day. See usually what we put in our mouths as our first meal or even a snack, is what you will follow. We tend to crave and follow that same eating pattern throughout the day.

This is true in general when it comes to food selections regardless to if a person is a faster or not. I mean think about it. If your first meal of the day is a steak and a good leafy green salad or a nice large omelet with side of fruit; (if you are hungry at all for another meal), you will likely choose something well balanced for the next meal. What this could look like is something rich in protein and a side of veggies to close out your feeding for the day.

This is because our palates tend to follow the pattern in which we have trained them. When we train the palate to eat healthier, we tend to crave the healthier food choices. When we train it to always reach for the salt, sugar & fat... it follows.

No stock piling-

When I choose to have dessert, I'm actually careful about what I choose and where I get it from. For example, I've learned its better for me to get a quick slice of cake from the grocery store bakery vs baking a whole cake. The temptation to eat the cake daily (until it's gone) is starring me in the face. So purchasing the slice, enjoying it and getting it out of my system, gives me better results.

I could also reach for my go to desserts - the piece of orange-chocolate or my prepare my berry dessert.

Its the same for me when I crave potato chips. My favorite flavor is salt & vinegar kettle chips. Its a wise decision for me just to drive to the store and buy a small personal bag of chips vs buying the large bag to be kept in the house for a few days to munch on. However a great fasting tip is to use a little Pink Himalayan salt on the tongue. Enjoy the flavor in your mouth for a few seconds and the craving goes away! I promise you it works. There were many times that I was able to say No to junk food because I had my pink salt handy.

See although I was fasting daily and could eat anything I wanted in my feeding window... I had to remember the results I was trying to achieve. And since certain foods were triggers for me; eating them often would lead me to relapsing into my old habits.

Its like we are waking up the beast when we keep running back too often to the foods that made us fat to begin with. The question is - are we willing to retrain our palates to eat nutrient dense foods for example kale, salmon, or maybe shellfish? Or are we going to continue to answer when the cravings come knocking?

While continuing to clean the house that morning; I pondered the consequences of eating that much sugar in the morning. The more I thought about the consequences, the less desirable the cup-cake became to me. Besides - if I gave in, that would be day two of splurging and that was just not going to work!

Remember how far you've come

Most importantly I reflected on where I had come from and how I had to discipline myself to fast every day.

A plunder of thoughts from my past begin to hit me. I remembered the times I would sit in the grocery store parking lot and eat half the bag of salt and vinegar chips (the family size bag) before I got home because of the stressful work day. I thought about my earlier years of failing when I was religiously buying the two cinnamon fry doughnuts every morning before work. The truth is, I was addicted to junk food prior to adapting to fasting and I just didn't want to go backwards.

So as a result, I dismissed the second day of splurging and I won the battle in my head and crushed the cravings that were trying to invade my taste buds! I fasted that day as I did every other day in my process and was proud of myself for not giving in.

Its important that we don't lose focus on our goals. If you are reading this chapter and you have already met your goal or even if you're not quite there yet; maintaining your weight loss success is just as important as you initially dropping the pounds. Think about it; you've made it this far and you can't allow frequent splurging or binging to derail your success. As discussed in the fasting chapter, you can eat what you like in your feeding window. Its your party, your journey. We may find that we just have to delay that treat until your feeding window versus denying yourself totally. In my case - regarding the cupcake, I had already had a day of splurging and did not need a second one the very next day. So sometimes we must tell ourselves **No** depending on the circumstance. Remember… this journey is all about balance.

I'd like to share some strategies that I still put into practice to ensure that I **"Avoid Relapse"** in my fasting lifestyle.

Stick to the plan-

By now you have probably figured out which foods you like and don't like; as well as what foods work for you and which don't. Establishing a pattern of consistency insures we are successful and keeps us on track.

For instance, you have probably determined which fasting schedule works for you in-spite of how busy your life is. So don't be tempted to deviate from it because you have seen some success on the scale and the way your clothes fit. **We can't become comfortable and let our guards down just because we have made it, or we're almost there.** This causes me to think about addiction overall. I also think of my son walking through his own addiction process. He sometimes would feel like he could handle things on his own and would begin going back to the friends that he started the bad habits with or going back to the places that caused the triggers to come alive again in his life.

So take the time to create your own meal plans of foods you like to eat that are good for you nutritiously.

There is nothing like preparation! **Know what you are going to eat and when you're going to eat it!** Also, if you know you're facing a busy day, cook your meal ahead of time and have it ready so you only have to warm it up. If you are unable to do this, at least prep the meal - you know… cut up the veggies ahead of time, season the meat the night before. You will set yourself up for failure if you think you can fast for 16 hours plus and not have a clue of what you're going to eat in your feeding window. And trust me, running to the drive-thru too often, you will find to be expensive and counterproductive of what you're trying to achieve.

I worked from home when I started fasting, so I would prep for my first meal at 6:30 or 7:00am when I got up. I generally ate bacon and eggs for my first meal and I would cook the bacon in the morning although I was not going to eat it until the afternoon. If I wanted boiled eggs, I would boil them while the bacon was cooking. However, if I had a taste for cheese eggs, I would wait until a few minutes before my feeding window to scramble them. Same practice for my last meal of the day, I would brine and season the meat I was going to grill. If I was having salad or hot veggies for that meal, I would prepare ahead of my feeding window so I was not sabotaging my results by grabbing the first piece of food I saw when my fasting window ended. Remember, chances are if you do not live alone, there will be junk food in the house - and its usually someone else's junk food; but you have to be prepared not to succumb to it because you didn't prepare.

I also learned to prepare by taking food with me if I knew I was not going to be home during my feeding window. Sometimes I would grab a quick salad while I was out but there were times, I would take food with me to eat. For instance, the second time I went to see my new hair braider, I took food with me since I knew the appointment would be long. I also found a wonderful gem online that allowed me to reheat my food while in my car! Yes, it plugs into the cigarette lighter and heats up your food quickly. It looks like a small tool box so its very compact. It has to be used when the car is not in motion. However, a meal can be heated in a manner of minutes. This is also a great resource to have when traveling longer distances so you stay on track with your meal goals. That wonderful gem is called RoadPro portable stove and can be found at different retailers online.

Continue to stay Active-

Skipping a workout here or there because of a busy schedule is expected in this journey but If you've reached your goal and looking at your thinner frame in the mirror and thinking you no longer have to exercise; you're going to face failure and disappointment. It is imperative that we stay active to maintain the weight loss. When I first started going to the gym in my early days, I would actually scratch my head at all the thin women in my class and wonder why they were there and so diligent about showing up?

They were there because the wanted to stay thin! I even see some of them in my local grocery store today, several years later and they look the same.

We have got to keep the same disciplines in place that aided us in loosing the weight to insure that we maintain the weight loss.

As mentioned, you may have to switch things up, try a new routine or rediscover an outdoor activity to make exercise fun and exciting. Join a volleyball or a soccer league. We are never too old to stay active and trust me, as you drop the pounds you will notice how much more energy you will have. It inspires and encourages me when I see women and men that are older than me in my local area out biking, walking and running. It reminds me that regardless to age - we have to keep moving in order to keep moving. We improve our strength and balance and are less prone to injury when we make exercise a priority.

Personally at this point in my journey, since I have dropped the pounds, my current goal is to dig deeper into weight lifting to gain more lean muscle. While I did lift some while dropping the pounds; I'd like to take it to the next level by working with my husband or a trainer so that I use proper form while lifting.

So we've got to make the decision that we're making a lifestyle change vs a temporary solution to lose weight.

Coping in High-Risk Situations-

You will find rather quickly as I did that you can't just let your hair down as you move forward. You have to always be aware of what you're eating especially in certain environments.

High risk situations can easily cause us to deviate from our plan if we aren't focused on where we're trying to go. Some examples of these environments can be the movie theater, dinner with friends, an event such as a buffet dinner party; or even a season of the year. Personally, vacations and holidays were high-risk for me especially in my early days of fasting. What worked for me was to do OMAD on those special occasion days and enjoy the same foods as everyone else but deciding to limit my portion size when I did eat. As I write to you today, Thanksgiving is approaching and I will definitely do OMAD on the holiday and even a few days after as I enjoy the left overs. My dear friends, this lifestyle is sustainable and I promise you, as you make your own personal commitment to consistently fast and exercise; handling high-risk situations become easier.

If a high-risk time for you is dining with friends or family I encourage you to plan ahead prior to the event. Be sure and preview the restaurant's menu online before arriving. Also be prepared to cut your portion sizes by asking for a take out box if the portions served are too large. There were also events that I attended while I was actually in my fasting window and I chose to hang out, laugh and enjoy the evening and only have water. My mind was made up and I couldn't allow anyone or event to derail my results.

Also prepare yourself mentally when dining with family or friends especially if you're at a point to where your weight loss is noticeable to others. Some will criticize what you choose to eat. Some will make negative comments about your success if they know you are practicing intermittent fasting. I encourage you to stay focused and even plan your response ahead of time as to how you're going to respond to them verbally. As I write this chapter this morning, I am attending a wedding later today and there will be many people there that I haven't seen in a long time; but I plan to smile and respond in a positive way if I am greeted with negative comments or snide remarks about my weight loss. Better yet, I am prepared for the ones that just look you up and down but say nothing.

I can recall one year when I was on the upside of my weight loss journey over hearing my aunt say to my cousin - "Look at Faith, she looks good, she's not as fat as she used to be". Of course, I kept a smile on my face as I heard my precious aunt say this. Heck!.. I was sitting less than ten feet away from her. So its imperative that you be proactive and plan how and when you're going to eat as well as plan your response to the negativity that will come.

Maintain your Supportive Network

Remain Present - Continue to stay connected to the people or groups that helped you reach goal. If we fall or slip up, it's easy to feel ashamed and to isolate ourselves. But reaching out when you've messed up is crucial in getting back on track. Its also good to be honest and vocal when you feel like you're going to relapse back into the old behaviors. Its OK to be honest and say… "I don't want to work out today" Or "today, I don't want to fast". "Today, I just want to eat when I want and whatever I want". It's in the moments that we choose to share our vulnerability with our real supporters, that we receive a genuine push or word of encouragement to stay on track. In my online fasting group, I would read post daily from women that were on the verge of giving up, or post from women that had fallen off the wagon. Others in the group were quick to offer words of encouragement, tips or strategies to get back on track, or just deciding to be that woman's cheerleader to keep her motivated. Friends, we have the tools we need to lose the weight and maintain it without the use of potions, pills, tricks and gimmicks from corporations trying to sell us the next big lie for weight loss success.

Participation time:

In the space provided below:

I'd like for you to think about your triggers, what are some triggers that could send you back to your old habits? Which environments do you need to avoid or curtail? How will you use the strategies in this chapter to insure you don't relapse or sabotage your success?

_____

_____

_____

_____

_____

_____

_____

_____

14.

A charge to share

DEAD AT 36! The phone rang one afternoon and the information received on the other end of the line made my heart sink. We had gotten news that a young man my husband and I mentored in our church youth group had passed away. I think I was just stunned the entire day and could only think of his family. It had been many years since we had seen him but to hear of his passing was shocking. My questions were how and why? How could someone many years younger than us be gone? Someone we watched as a teenager laugh and joke with his friends at church.

I learned that he passed from complications of diabetes. As a teen he was sort of on the husky side; but you just never thought that the fact the he was a little overweight would lead to an early death. Most of his young adult life he suffered from diabetes and eventually lead to kidney failure and then to his demise. I just wept that day in disbelief. The news also made me take self-inventory as I think we all do when we hear of someone passing due to health complications; especially young adults. The family friend I mentioned in an earlier chapter that passed away from a stroke still bothers me today because she was only 29 or 30 years old. To clarify she had a series of strokes and a heart attack and then her organs shut down. She was gone within a week of being rushed to the emergency room.

The phrase that we've heard about high blood pressure being the silent killer is absolutely true and we can't ignore the numbers. First, we have to our numbers. It's imperative that we check our blood pressure on a regular basis and do something about it if its high. It's important that we know our glucose numbers especially if we are diabetics.

Reality Check-

As I hear of family or friends that are receiving diagnosis at a rapid pace of diabetes, high blood pressure and those having heart attacks; it really concerns me. First, I feel a sense of sadness for the person and then I feel a little scared because it could have been me receiving the diagnosis. I also think of a friend that has multiple health issues going on in her body. We don't talk often but when we do; it seems that I find out about a new ailment. One thing I know for sure is that death has no age limit and we have to live our lives knowing that we only get this one body to care for.

As I go about my everyday life and observe people that are struggling with obesity and achieving better health; it sparks my attention because I care. I often wonder what their story is? How did they get to the to the point to receive a certain diagnosis from their physicians? How did he get to the place to where he can barely walk? Or why is that he or she has to take a plethora of medications each day? I don't wonder or ponder these things in judgment but out of genuine concern for my brothers and sisters in life. This concern impels me share with others how I've been able to lose 50 pounds.

It impels me to share how it is that I look and feel younger than I did years ago. While I have learned to temper my passion about this fasting lifestyle; I never pass up an opportunity to share my experiences and how fasting works with those that genuinely inquire. See you will have many that will want to know how you lost the weight but when you tell them through fasting and making better food choices, they may be quickly turned off. This is because many simply don't want to do the work or make the sacrifice it takes to reverse old behaviors. However, just because some may be turned off and actually ridicule you for fasting, you can't let that stop you. Always be willing to share with those that are interested. Personally, I see it as a responsibility, a charge to share. A charge to help someone make a change for the better.

Why I Share-

The grocery store experience-

I share how fasting has changed my life because sometimes, I am brought to tears or have a deep burden for the welfare of others I encounter. I recall being in the grocery store one Saturday just doing my normal shopping. As I was on a particular isle I saw a couple both in the motorized scooter carts coming up the aisle. My first thought was Wow! They both have a difficulty walking. I couldn't help but notice that they were severely overweight and one was following slowly behind the other up the isle.

Eventually, they came to a stop and it was right in front of the candy. The wife was struggling to reach for the candy from her scooter. One of the bags of candy fell from the shelf onto the floor and her husband came over to assist her. His form of assisting her was to push the candy more in her reach with the cane he had. I watched almost in disbelief as they stocked her basket with several packages and varieties of candy. I then glanced at the husband's cart and his was full of packs of can soda. Honestly, my heart ached as I continued to shop. I was just baffled at how we as mankind have become slaves to the sugar crave. I mean to be barely walking and need to use a scooter to shop but still buying the crap that has gotten us in that condition can be plaguing. But its only plaguing or mind boggling once you've made the switch. One you're on the outside looking in - then it's shocking. Because when I was buying the 2 cinnamon fry doughnuts as my breakfast 5 days a week; I didn't see anything wrong with it either. The gooey cinnamon doughnuts were at least 500 calories each and that was just my breakfast. Yep, my first meal of the day was just straight -up soft, fluffy sugar! So as I encounter incidences like my grocery store experience, I feel impelled to help anyone that's willing to start making changes in their lives.

Thanksgiving - the all-time high

My family always gathers at Thanksgiving just as many families do all over the country. We had our usual spread of the traditional foods and a large variety of desserts. I recall this particular gathering vividly because it was a year that I had lost some weight and was feeling good in the outfit I wore that year to the gathering. (Yep, I'm a little vain!) Personally, I was very conscience not to over eat because it was just one of the seasons in my life that I was really trying to do better about my health. All of my family had eaten and many were gathering around the desserts. I was busy socializing with everyone and I happen to glance at one of my brothers. He was sitting in a rocking chair and the look on his face was all too familiar. He had the same look I would often have when I over ate.

He didn't have to tell me how he was feeling. I knew his blood pressure was high and he just looked disoriented. I asked him if he was OK and he slowly said he was alright. I didn't pressure him but I knew he wasn't feeling good. I wasn't sure if he had skipped his blood pressure pill that morning or what but I was genuinely concerned about him. I wondered if we would need to take him to the hospital. He remained quiet for the remainder of the day and just rested in the chair. I could only imagine what his blood pressure may have been if we had taken it that day.

See that was all too familiar to me because during the years that I would ignore the fact that I had high blood pressure; I would still sit and over eat knowing I would eventually feel better.

I was literally playing "Russian Roulette" with my life! My dear brothers and sisters, we simply cannot to continue to ignore our blood pressure and our A1C levels just hoping things will get better. Our health simply isn't going to improve if we don't start to take action. Just as I've mentioned, death has no age limit and many parents in their late 40's and early 50's are burying their 20- and 30-year-old children; due to their declined health issues. See it's not longer just the gang violence or flying stray bullets that are killing our young adults today. Its the chronic addiction to sugar, processed foods, over-eating and bad relationships with food that's killing our loved ones. As I conclude this book our world as we know it; is currently in a pandemic where many have suffered and died from a virus coined as COVID-19.

We have seen just as many young adults pass away from COVID-19 (if not more); just as the elderly have passed. What we learned about Covid is that many people with weak immune systems were hugely at risk regardless to age. This hit home for us personally with one of my husband's cousins. As a matter of fact, this cousin is the son of his cousin that I mentioned earlier in the book. The female relative that passed away from her health challenges; the one that was the same age as me. Now several years later, her 24-year-old son that is a diabetic contracts COVID-19 and passes away. My God! How could this be?

So ladies and gentlemen, once we learn and do better, we have a charge, we have a responsibility to share and help educate others. This doesn't mean we have to be weird by trying to shove it down the throats of our family and friends. But just live the life and as people inquire or if the opportunity arises, take the open door and discuss how fasting and making healthier choices has changed your life. Please, don't be that over bearing person that criticizes everyone for what is on their plates at gatherings. You will soon notice that people cringe when you show up or begin to exclude you from the invite list. We have to remember in our sharing that we all are on different levels and phases of our lives and you can't expect more from people than what they've been exposed to.

The next generation-

Parents, we have a responsibility to teach and help our children. Especially if you are raising small children. If your children are minors, you definitely have the ability to decide what they eat.

Yes! You do! - Because you buy the groceries. The earlier that we start our children with making healthy food choices the better. It really saddens me to see a family - a dad, a mom with the children trailing behind and the entire family is severely obese. See this over indulgence is not prejudice to any particular race. This is a widespread issue throughout our western society.

If we can begin to train our children's taste buds from birth - this thing is doable! I often think of one of my nieces. My sister-in-law fed her home made baby food from the time she was able to eat solid food. She barely knew what commercial baby food taste like. She was primarily fed home-made whole food! Her mom would blend up fresh broccoli or fresh squash she had prepared for her baby. This natural whole food was free of salt, sugar and other preservatives. She would occasionally eat organic baby food (free from GMO's) if her mother may not have time to prepare something. Currently my niece is a healthy vibrant five-year-old that was hardly ever ill as a baby. It amazes me to see her sit and eat a plate of raw bell peppers or raw broccoli. So it is possible. Even if your children didn't have a start like this, it's possible to reverse the gobs of processed foods and sugar we are allowing our kids to eat. This can be done little by little so its not such a drastic change for your family.

Don't be pressured

I encourage you not be pressured by screaming toddlers and adolescents that are demanding the junk food over the healthier choices you are endeavoring to introduce to your family. Be willing to be patient with the process and the more they see you practice healthy habits, they will follow. My sons are now in their early twenties and are becoming more health conscience about what they eat, especially since they have seen me adapt a fasting life style. One of them moved back home temporarily and mentioned how I only seem to cook "healthier food" now. This definitely was not the case when they were growing up. They were eating the fried chicken from the box a couple times a week just like me because it's what I bought and put on the plate in front of them. If we are consistent with changing what we serve our families especially our children, we are retraining their taste buds just as we had to do for ourselves. It's about flipping the switch.

Permission to indulge-

For many of us we were granted to permission to over eat believe it or not at CHURCH! Yes, I said it! Especially if you grew up in the South; soul food was served in an abundance. I'm sure like me; you can remember the countless after - church dinners on special Sundays. There were also bake sales or fish fry's to support a particular ministry at church.

And for a lot of us, there didn't have to be a special occasion, we would often gather as friends at local restaurants or dining out was a Friday night pass time after church service. So although we couldn't seem to do much socially, there seem to be no problem with loading our plates and just overeating together. Although my father was a tall slender man that was careful about what he ate; many of his preacher colleagues were quite the opposite. I can still envision the overweight robust men dressed in fancy suits with bellies as big as Santa. For me there was a lot that we were forbidden to do because just about everything was considered a sin or just down right worldly. But the gluttony that went on was OK! As a kid I didn't seem to notice but I eventually learned the women who looked as if they were stuffed in the dresses they were wearing were battling high blood pressure and diabetes.

And the funerals of church members we attended (or mainly our parents) were practically premature deaths from chronic health issues.

Hoarding

For many years in a church I attended, I was the hospitality department head which meant I was responsible for planning a menu and overseeing the serving of our pastors and special guest after certain church events.

My team and I were feeding these ministers as late at 10 or 11pm at night. At the request of the pastor, we were usually serving soul food and an array of decedent deserts.

I would also be asked to pack up plates for guest that hadn't even finished their meals yet!

The packing of plates or hoarding as I like to call it was a common thing at church events or even family gathering.

While leftovers are expected, sometimes it was an awful site to see as people scrambled around the table or kitchen to pack up food as if there was no tomorrow!

Share by teaching

I mentioned earlier that I am a preacher's kid and grew up going to church several times a week. As I matured and began to see death occur more rapidly in our churches, I began to realize there was an imbalance in the teaching. Although we teach and encourage growth in our relationships with God; we can't leave out the importance of taking care of our physical temples. We can't just scurry past our health because its not spiritual enough. What we eat, and how much we move is just as important of how much we love God and how well we are to treat our neighbors. I believe health and fitness should be discussed or at least mentioned in pulpits all across America.

I'm not saying is has to be the Pastor or the leader of the church that shares how we can live healthier lives; but be open to having some one experienced in your church to teach and help the members. Another option is to bring someone in to do a seminar on health and wellness. We have to start to care for our bodies just as well as we take care of our spirit man. Remember we are made up of soul, body and spirit. If our physical bodies are broken down and in shambles, how much work can we really do for the Kingdom of God? If preachers are stroking out or having heart attacks in the pulpit today - what does that say about us - the church? To me it says, we can believe God for change in our lives in every area except for our health. We just simply don't want to do the work and that saddens me. However, there is hope! We can make changes in our health and share it with others. Remember, we are our brother's keeper.

This brings me to the reason I decided to write this book. I felt a strong responsibility to share my experiences with a desire to help others. I believe that we should help others and pull them along once we have succeeded in something.

It breaks my heart to hear of family or friends that are suffering greatly in their bodies because of chronic illnesses. It's my desire to help as many people as I can change their thinking and behavior about food and exercise. I would love to see us all live healthier lives. I'd like to see diabetes, kidney and heart disease reversed through better nutritional habits and being more active. I'd like to see kids and teens take charge of their health early in life so that they don't reach adulthood and experience the same health problems their parents may have experienced.

I mentioned in a previous chapter that there were several people that planted the seed of exercise and healthy eating in my life.

Although it took a while for the seed to manifest fruit because I wasn't ready to consistently do the work, it finally clicked for me. When I got tired of the Doctor changing my blood pressure medication to get my pressure to normal levels; I made the decision to so something about it. When I was tired of the belly aches and being fat year after year; I took charge of my own life and I wouldn't trade it for anything in the world! So since making the switch, I can't keep it to myself. I've noticed sometimes as women when we make progress in life; we can often keep it to ourselves in a selfish manner. But no ma'am, no sir! We have a responsibility to share, a responsibility to help. Again, its about finding balance with how we help and share but we must be willing to share because someone's health or maybe even their life depends on it.

So after reading this book I hope that you have a better understanding of how to make the switch from poor eating habits to healthier habits as well as making a commitment to be more active. **It is my prayer that you come to the realization that you no longer have to be a slave to your cravings.** It is my hope that you will embark on this wonderful journey of fasting to meet your weight loss goal as well as reap the other benefits of fasting.

I hope you are fired up and ready for this to be your last time on the Fat Merry-Go-Round. I hope you're tired of circling around the same issue year after year just as I was. I pray this is the time you finally say enough is enough and I'm ready to make permanent change.

As you make this commitment for yourself and start to see your health improve; I want to encourage you to share what you have learned as well as your own experiences with someone else.

So as the compliments flow in about how great you look and your weight loss success; don't be selfish. Pull someone out of the fire!

We all have a charge to share!

Works Cited

n.d. *6 Popular Ways to Do Intermittent Fasting.* Accessed March 8, 2021. https://www.healthline.com/nutrition/6-ways-to-do-intermittent-fasting.

n.d. *Autophagy: What You Need to Know.* Accessed March 8, 2021. https://www.healthline.com/health/autophagy.

Babar Shahzad MD, MSc, BSc. n.d. *The Real Deal About Liquid Fasting.* Accessed March 8, 2021. https://dofasting.com/blog/liquid-fasting/.

2017. *Beware High Levels of Cortisol, the Stress Hormone.* February 5. Accessed March 8, 2021. https://www.premierhealth.com/your-health/articles/women-wisdom-wellness-/beware-high-levels-of-cortisol-the-stress-hormone.

n.d. *Circadian rhythm.* Accessed March 8, 2021. https://en.wikipedia.org/wiki/Circadian_rhythm.

2019. *Diabetes and the Body.* January 15. Accessed March 8, 2021. https://www.diabetes.co.uk/body/.

2019. *Does Intermittent Fasting Work?* March 13. Accessed March 8, 2021. https://healthtalk.unchealthcare.org/does-intermittent-fasting-work/.

2020. *Getting past a weight-loss plateau.* February 25. Accessed March 8, 2021. https://www.mayoclinic.org/healthy-lifestyle/weight-loss/in-depth/weight-loss-plateau/art-20044615.

n.d. *Glands & Hormones A-Z.* Accessed March 8, 2021. https://www.hormone.org/your-health-and-hormones/glands-and-hormones-a-to-z.

2019. *Growth hormone, athletic performance, and aging.* June 19. Accessed March 8, 2021. https://www.health.harvard. edu/diseases-and-conditions/growth-hormone-athletic-performance-and-aging.

Helen Kollias, PhD, John Berardi, PhD, CSCS. n.d. *The surprising problem with calorie counting. [Infographic].* Accessed March 8, 2021. https://www.precisionnutrition.com/ problem-with-calorie-counting-calories-out.

n.d. *Hormones.* Accessed March 8, 2021. https://www.yourhormones. info/hormones/.

n.d. *I Tried Extreme Fasting by Eating Once a Day — Here's What Happened.* Accessed March 8, 2021. https://www.healthline.com/ health/food-nutrition/one-meal-a-day-diet.

Ives, Laurel. 2018. *Can the science of autophagy boost your health?* May 6. Accessed March 8, 2021. https://www.bbc.com/news/ health-44005092.

Kabala, Jillian. 2018. *Intermittent Fasting and Keto: Should You Combine the Two?* November 5. Accessed March 8, 2021. https:// www.healthline.com/nutrition/intermittent-fasting-and-keto.

Link, Rachel. 2018. *8 Health Benefits of Fasting, Backed by Science.* July 30. Accessed March 8, 2021. https://www.healthline.com/nutrition/ fasting-benefits.

Myers, Bryan. 2019. *What Are the Benefits of a Liquid Fast?* July 17. Accessed March 8, 2021. https://www.livestrong.com/ article/446251-what-are-the-benefits-of-a-liquid-fast.

Nunez, Kirsten. 2019. *Everything You Want to Know About Dry Fasting.* October 30. Accessed March 8, 2021. https://www.healthline.com/ health/food-nutrition/dry-fasting.

n.d. *Short History of Fasting.* Accessed March 8, 2021. https://www. targethealth.com/post/short-history-of-fasting.

Tello, Monique. 2020. *https://www.health.harvard.edu/blog/intermittent-fasting-surprising-update-2018062914156.* February 10. Accessed

March 8, 2021. https://www.health.harvard.edu/blog/intermittent-fasting-surprising-update-2018062914156.

n.d. *The Warrior Diet: Review and Beginner's Guide.* Accessed March 8, 2021. https://www.healthline.com/nutrition/warrior-diet-guide.

healthline.com/nutrition/6-ways-to-do-intermittent-fasting.

n.d. *I Tried Extreme Fasting by Eating Once a Day — Here's What Happened.* Accessed March 8, 2021. https://www.healthline.com/health/food-nutrition/one-meal-a-day-diet.

n.d. *The Warrior Diet: Review and Beginner's Guide.* Accessed March 8, 2021. https://www.healthline.com/nutrition/warrior-diet-guide.

CPSIA information can be obtained
at www.ICGtesting.com
Printed in the USA
LVHW051300300621
691545LV00015B/1265

9 781662 817014